THE ACCOUNTABILITY OF BIOETHICS COMMITTEES AND CONSULTANTS

SIGRID FRY-REVERE, JD, PhD

Frederick 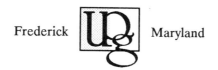 Maryland

University Publishing Group Inc.
Frederick, Maryland 21701

ISBN 1-55572-012-9

Preface and Acknowledgments

In the Karen Quinlan case of 1976, the New Jersey Supreme Court suggested that the hospital refer cessation of life support issues to a bioethics committee to help incompetent patients' doctors and families make their decisions. Since 1976 the use of bioethics committees and consultants has greatly increased. Recommendations for the establishment of bioethics committees by the President's Commission for the Study of Ethical Problems in Medicine and Biomedical and Behavioral Research in 1983 and the Department of Health and Human Services in 1984 precipitated a rapid increase in their use. Although it is uncertain what percentage of medical facilities have bioethics consultants, estimates of the percentage of institutions with bioethics committees have grown from between one and sixteen percent to between sixty and ninety percent in the past ten years. One state, Maryland, has even mandated the use of such committees and Congress considered, but rejected, a similar mandate during the 1990 session. Although bioethics committees and consultants vary in the functions they perform, their impact on medical decision making cannot be ignored.

One important question that must be addressed, given the ever growing use of bioethics committees and consultants, is whether they should be held accountable for their advice and, if so, how and to whom they should be held accountable. The concept of accountability used throughout this book has a very narrow and specific sense. It is not accountability in the moral sense of doing the right thing or achieving the "good," but rather a concept from legal or political philosophy that stresses process over content. Bioethics consultation is no longer theoretical, and some effort must be made to discuss how, if at all, those engaged in such consultation should be regulated.

With issues as important as life and death decisions in the balance, some options for holding bioethics committees and consultants accountable for their advice should be explored. The uncertainties common to bioethical dilemmas and the pluralist nature of our society make the regulation of the content of bioethics advice unacceptable; however, mechanisms that encourage a uniformly fair process of granting and conducting bioethics consultations are needed. While the debate over what is right in the medical context continues, we should at least try to ensure that the questions being faced are handled in an acceptable fashion.

Once the case for accountability has been made (part 1), existing mechanisms for ensuring accountability are examined (parts 2 and 3). Those mechanisms are then evaluated for their applicability to bioethics committees and consultants (part 4).

This book does not reconsider the well-documented debate over the need for bioethics committees and consultants and their proper functions. The ever growing use of bioethics committees and consultants is justification enough for a discussion of what should be done to ensure that bioethics consultations are handled in a procedurally fair manner. The goals of bioethics consultation will be briefly discussed in chapter 2, where questions such as whether bioethics committees and consultants should make binding decisions or only give advice, whether they should primarily educate or set institutional policy, and whether they should primarily facilitate communication or advocate certain moral principles will be considered.

I begin my inquiry by examining alternative theories of accountability, rejecting all but the one I call a theory of "social accountability." The particular type of social accountability at issue in this book functions through social mechanisms such as professional organizations, court-enforced liability, and government regulations that require a certain process to be followed, but not through mechanisms of moral accountability, such as acting in good conscience or in accordance with particular philosophical or religious beliefs intended to dictate the content of advice. I explore the philosophical boundaries of this notion of accountability and lay a foundation to justify holding bioethics committees and consultants accountable.

The advantages of providing accountability for bioethics committees and consultants are too great to ignore. There must be a way to encourage a consistent process for initiating bioethics consultations and for well-considered resolution of the very difficult bioethical questions that arise in the medical context.

The next step in my investigation is to analyze five types of existing mechanisms for the implementation of accountability that may be applicable to bioethics consultation. In particular, I will look at professional self-regulation, licensure and professional discipline, government contracting, judicial remedies, and government commissions. Then I will discuss the applicability of these standards to bioethics committees and consultants.

I conclude that holding bioethics committees and consultants accountable for the advice they give would help make the granting and conducting of bioethics consultations more equitable. First, questions of how accountability should be ensured need to be studied by government commissions and/or professional organizations. Then, the results of such studies should be implemented through professional self-regulation and/or government regulation.

And finally, a potential for court review, if necessary, should not be precluded. Some specifics of how bioethics committees and consultants should be regulated are discussed. Issues such as access to consultation services, adequate training for committees and consultants, consultation proceedings, documentation, peer review, appeal procedures, and committee composition should be considered by those developing specific requirements for holding bioethics committees and consultants accountable for their advice.

In closing, I wish to express my loving appreciation to Bob, Nathan, and Ian for understanding my need to spend so much time preparing this book and my heartfelt gratitude to LeRoy Walters, Terry Pinkard, and Judith Areen for their guidance.

CONTENTS

PART THREE
THE ACCOUNTABILITY OF INSTITUTIONAL COMMITTEES

PART ONE

Why Bioethics Committees and Consultants Should Be Held Accountable for Their Advice

Introduction to Part One

Part 1 will establish a philosophical foundation for the analysis and the conclusions of parts to come. The presupposition of any analysis of accountability mechanisms is that accountability is desirable. This part will explain why holding bioethics committees and consultants accountable is justifiable and advantageous both from a public policy perspective and the perspective of the bioethics profession itself. Chapter 1 defines the concept of accountability as it is used throughout this book, clearly distinguishing between those types of moral accountability that concentrate on how we can hold individuals accountable for their actions, and those forms of social accountability that are more concerned with who is to be held accountable to whom, for what, and why. Then, chapter 2, relying on various aspects of social and political theory, argues that accountability in the form of procedural due process is critical to the proper functioning and success of bioethics consultation.

CHAPTER ONE

A Philosophical Analysis
of the Concept of Accountability

Choosing a Theory of Accountability

Discovering the Accountability Equation

Accountability, in common parlance, means to be obliged to give satisfactory reasons for one's actions, to be capable of giving an explanation for one's actions, to be responsible for one's conduct, to be made to pay for one's conduct, or to reckon with the consequences of one's actions.[1] The philosophical consideration of this concept and the related concept of *responsibility* has occupied the attention of philosophers for millennia.

Responsibility, in its broadest sense, not only includes one's intentional conduct, but also anything with which one is seen to have a causal relationship (whether this perception is justifiable or not), including moral character, physical and psychological characteristics, salvation, and even unintentional effects on one's own life or the lives of others. Most philosophical discussions of responsibility, however, concentrate on actions or consequences over which individuals do, or should, exercise control. Theories of responsibility are often analyzed in action theory,[2] ethics,[3] theology,[4] and legal or political philosophy.[5]

Of particular interest in this book is one aspect of responsibility--namely, the relationship between the responsible person and the agent holding him or her responsible. Although many philosophers distinguish this type of responsibility from others, they do not necessarily term it accountability. In the interest of working with clearly defined terms, this book will always refer to this particular aspect of responsibility theory as accountability.

Most theories of accountability seek to decipher some aspect of one of two equations: (1) a person, X, is accountable for his or her actions if X acted freely or intentionally and X's action or inaction is causally related to the outcome for which X is being held accountable; or (2) a person, group of persons, or institution, W, is held accountable by X for Y because Z.

Moral and Social Accountability

Theories of Moral Accountability

Moral theories of accountability concentrate on the first of these equations: A person, X, is accountable for his or her actions if X acted freely or intentionally and X's action or inaction is causally related to the outcome for which X is being held accountable.[6] In their attempt to explain this equation, many philosophers have considered in one form or another the essential questions: What are voluntary action,[7] intention,[8] and freedom?[9] Other relevant questions include: How do mind and body interact to make something willed a reality?[10] How do we determine which consequences a person should be held accountable for in the long chain of events that can result from one act of will?[11] Most of these issues deal with one aspect or another of the simple question: "*How* can we hold anyone accountable for his or her actions?" While the resolution of this question is required before any theory of accountability can be developed, it is not itself a discussion of the accountability relationship between a responsible person and the agent holding him or her responsible.

Once the potential for moral accountability is established, some moral theories do address the accountability relationship, but they tend to emphasize accountability to oneself or a higher being.[12] Although this and the earlier mentioned questions of moral accountability are universally applicable to all human beings, they are not uniquely relevant to bioethics committees and consultants. In the interest of concentrating on issues of accountability that will provide practical guidance for bioethics committees and consultants, this book assumes that human beings are free to act and cause events for which they are directly responsible and that some form of internal mechanism of accountability, whether based on conscience or belief, is essential to human interaction. These assumptions allow me to concentrate on the external mechanisms of accountability that are unique to bioethics committees and consultants.

Theories of Social Accountability

Social, or what is also called legal, accountability deals with the second equation mentioned above: A person, group of persons or institution, W, is held accountable by X for Y because Z. Theories of social accountability also consider questions of free will[13] and causation,[14] but they more frequently concentrate on "*Who* is to be held accountable by *whom*, for *what* and *why*?" When this question is addressed by political or legal philosophers, the accountability relationship considered is generally not one between a responsible agent and his or her own conscience or a higher being, but rather between the responsible person and government,[15] law,[16] or other social institutions.[17] An analysis of theories addressing what social mechanisms should be used to assure accountability could help solve some of the problems facing bioethics committees and consultants today.

Unfortunately, bioethics committees and consultants are in a unique situation, and many of the theories of social accountability presently available do not directly address the concerns this book seeks to resolve. Many theories of social accountability deal with the accountability of governments to their people, considering questions of democratic theory;[18] distributive justice;[19] or legislative, executive, or judicial responsiveness to the needs of the people.[20] Since bioethics committees and consultants are not government entities at the present time, these discussions are only tangentially relevant. Other common, but not directly related, issues considered by social theories of accountability are questions of punishment: "Why punish?"[21] "How should we punish?"[22] and "Which theory of punishment, deterrence, restitution, retribution, or rehabilitation is appropriate?"[23] Although discussion of what punishment, if any, is appropriate for what misconduct, is relevant to bioethics committees and consultants, this book will suggest the development of a before-the-fact[24] system of accountability that will provide guidance for bioethics committees and consultants before they act. Such before-the-fact guidance could help spare bioethics committees and consultants the costly and onerous development of standards through litigation. Consequently, this book discusses punishment only in so far as it assumes that a potential for sanctions is sometimes necessary for the enforcement of accountability.

An analysis of theories of social accountability proved most helpful in deciding on what basis holding bioethics committees and consultants accountable should be justified. This "why" aspect of the accountability equation is considered in the next chapter, where some possible justifications for holding bioethics committees and consultants accountable are explored. The justifications given rely on several alternative approaches, including appeals to reason, history, and shared cultural values.

Other aspects of the social accountability equation are also considered in other parts of this book. The goal of part 1 is to answer the "why" aspect of this accountability equation; it also addresses the "for what" question by discussing the nature and function of bioethics committees and consultants while obviating a need for constraints on the types of actions for which bioethics committees and consultants are held accountable. After part 1 addresses the "why" and "for what" aspects of the equation, parts 2 through 4 concentrate on the question of "by whom" bioethics committees and consultants should be held accountable.

Redefining Accountability

A Brief Definition

This book will use the term accountability in a very narrow and specific sense. Here, the meaning of accountability will be limited to social accountability, with the implication that there is some authoritative mechanism that has, as one of its goals, the maintenance of a degree of procedural fairness in how bioethics consultations are granted and conducted. These procedures must be implemented with integrity--they must be uniformly applied and consistently carried out. They must provide for equal access and an equality of process for like cases. Accountability does not regulate the content of advice but only the conditions under which that advice is given;[25] the accountability described here is concerned with process, not content. For accountability to exist, the mechanisms that assure procedural fairness should have the authority to impose sanctions when their procedures are not followed, but that ability is not necessitated by the definition of accountability. Nor must all mechanisms of accountability be concentrated in one institutional body; such mechanisms can consist of a combination of varied social forces.

Accountability and Responsibility

My use of the term accountability also implies that a failure to comply with a particular social process may have detrimental consequences. The detrimental consequence can be as insignificant as peer dissatisfaction or loss of one's membership in a private organization, or it can be as severe as loss of government licensure or court-imposed sanctions. For the most part, I am not interested in establishing sanctions for noncompliance with accountability standards but in devising a prescriptive system for guiding bioethics committees and consultants in their everyday functioning. The action that should be taken if members of bioethics committees or consultants act in an unacceptable manner--after-the-fact accountability--will not be the primary focus; the establishment of standards for their conduct--before-the-fact accountability--is central to my discussion.

Accountability requires a responsible actor, a party who receives advice, and a supervising agent or mechanism. The actors in this discussion are members of bioethics committees or bioethics consultants. The receiving parties are patients, their families, friends, and other surrogates or medical personnel. Who or what the supervising agent or mechanism should be is one of the questions this book seeks to answer.

Accountability as it is used here does not entail efforts to discourage erroneous decisions. In a new field like bioethics consultation, exactly what constitutes "good" or "correct" advice is debatable and makes ensuring correct advice an elusive task. Thus, the accountability discussed here is intended to encourage procedural fairness, rather than to evaluate decisions for their rightness or wrongness.

Accountability and Social Structures

The accountability at issue requires a structure imposed on or accepted by more than just one or two persons or entities. The structure is "social" because it is shared among those being held accountable. The decision of one bioethics consulting service to follow certain procedures may constitute a form of accountability, but such accountability is not relevant here. Nor are self-evaluative quality assurance programs[26] directly related to accountability. The mechanisms that assure accountability may require self-evaluation and certain quality assurance processes, but such procedures are not themselves mechanisms for assuring accountability. Rather, they represent the specific requirements a mechanism for assuring accountability may choose to implement. (chapter 10 discusses some of these specifics.) The procedural mechanisms I have in mind should help to assure client satisfaction, but that is not their primary purpose. The primary goal of accountability is a uniform process that helps to impose a structural fairness and predictability on how bioethics consultations are handled. The effective enforcement of accountability requires a widely applied system for assuring procedural fairness, not content regulation or the evaluation of programs in terms of client satisfaction.

Accountability is not based on principles of individual morality. Even if all members of a bioethics committee and all bioethics consultants were of impeccable moral character, society should still want to impose a procedural structure on how bioethics consultations are handled. Moral accountability is the responsibility we feel for our actions as judged by a higher being, the dictates of reason, or another source of our sense of right and wrong.[27] All moral accountability is internally motivated by conscience and belief. The accountability at issue in this book deals with the dictates established by society: the external, institutional controls our society has seen fit to place on human conduct.[28] Examples are government laws and regulation, rules of professional conduct, and peer pressure. Questions of moral accountability fall within the purview of ethics. Questions of social accountability, though sometimes dealt with in ethics, fall primarily within the purview of political or legal philosophy.

The social structures used to assure accountability may have their origins in either, or both, private or public sectors of society. Forms of private regulation could be as innocuous as common practices that become standards due to a general consensus regarding their appropriateness. These standards may become so accepted that peers frown on any deviation from the established practice. A private membership organization may impose certain criteria on its members or even hinge accreditation on the satisfaction of certain procedural requirements. More serious constraints on conduct could entail court-imposed sanctions or government regulation tied to licensure or funding.

The Nature of Accountability

Its Practical Nature

Accountability requires a functional mechanism, not some utopian ideal. The perfect structure or process for conducting bioethics consultations is not at issue here. Rather, my concern is the development of a "minimum floor" for what would be an acceptable process in our pluralistic society. By minimum floor, I mean a process that allows people who disagree to interact peaceably and come to some resolution without necessarily coming to a conclusion that everyone agrees is ethical. Such a process is far from perfect because it tolerates results that not all consider to be ethical, but it is functional in achieving peaceable resolutions of bioethical disputes in a pluralist society. Because some structures for assuring accountability may be better than others, parts 2 and 3 examine several existing systems of accountability for possible guidance in the realm of bioethics consultation.

Its Procedural Nature

The objective of accountability is not to regulate the content of bioethical advice, but rather to provide a system of procedural fairness that can function almost like a *Robert's Rules* for bioethics consultations. This approach avoids the need to debate the actual morality of certain outcomes yet interjects a modicum of fairness into what is now a very disorganized and unpredictable system for giving bioethical advice. The bioethics consulting services I know all differ in how they handle bioethics consultations. Some only allow medical staff to request consultations; some act in secrecy; some write opinions in patients' charts; some are composed purely of medical staff; and some only do after-the-fact review of cases rather than help clarify ethical issues during the decision-making process. A structural overlay that creates a uniformity in how bioethics consultations are handled would help assure equal access to bioethics consultation, create some predictability in how cases are handled, and provide some equality of treatment among cases heard.

H. Tristram Engelhardt, Jr., in his book *The Foundations of Bioethics*, argues that ethics itself, on the political level, should be procedural.[29] He argues that on the level of government ethics should, for the most part, prescribe how people interact without judging the rightness or wrongness of individual concepts of what is good.[30] Such a procedural ethic is the only way to resolve ethical disputes peaceably in a secular pluralist society.[31] I agree with Engelhardt's premise that, in a secular pluralist society, equitably applied procedures are critical to the peaceable resolution of ethical disputes; however, a goal of peaceful interaction is not enough to assure the fairness of procedures even if they are equitably applied. It is possible to promote peaceful interaction through unfair procedures, such as the threat of force or brainwashing. To avoid the conclusion that coercive methods are acceptable, philosophical limits must be placed on the procedural methods employed to promote peace. As will be discussed further in later sections, in addition to promoting peaceful interaction, procedures must be fair: they must respect individual choice and promote institutional integrity.

A system of fair procedures is the most constructive goal that the field of bioethics consultation can have until a social consensus is reached or government dictates what should be done regarding specific bioethical issues. As yet, bioethics committees and consultants do not, and perhaps they never should, have the authority to force individual action on ethical issues, particularly not on issues still unresolved by government or society.

Its Pluralist Nature

The accountability in question does not require justification for actions taken. It only requires evidence that proper procedures were followed. The procedures implemented to assure accountability may influence results, but they do not determine outcomes. Whether or not proper procedures were followed cannot be determined through an examination of outcomes. The social structures of due process should be fair; they must be based on a well-reasoned approach, but they should not require as part of the process that those giving advice justify their reasoning. For the most part, as far as accountability is concerned, if the prescribed process is followed, the outcome is acceptable even if some would argue with the reasoning used to justify the outcome. Principles of accountability are not violated if similar facts result in different advice.

Professional Accountability

Professionals generally are held accountable for the specific advice they give and are required to provide a rational justification for their advice based on the specific facts in question. This is a far more stringent type of accountability than what is being considered here. For bioethics consultation, there is no definite process for reasoning from specific facts to a specific conclusion. A doctor may be required to justify treating an uninjured arm, or an attorney may be required to justify advising an innocent person to confess to a crime he or she did not commit, but bioethics committees and consultants should not be required to provide justification for the advice they give. Unlike the case of the uninjured arm or the innocent client, there usually are no agreed-upon right or wrong answers in bioethics. Given the ethical diversities of a pluralist society, I cannot find a single set of facts that would necessitate a bioethics consultation to result in a specific conclusion. Albeit, in some areas the law, not an ethical consensus, has dictated certain conclusions (for example, abortion). Presently, therefore, there need only be a process for assuring that those engaged in bioethics consultations consider all the socially relevant factors.

Legal Versus Ethical Advice

Some might argue that, from a legal standpoint, our society has already placed some practical limits on the content of bioethical advice. It is possible that the advice a bioethics committee or consultant finds ethically appropriate, practically speaking, cannot be followed because the actions suggested are illegal. What is legal and what is ethical are not necessarily the same. Legal constraints on what can be done should not dictate the content of ethical advice; rather they should be weighed when considering the consequences of following that advice. A potential for legal retaliation does not necessarily make advice that is otherwise ethicial into bad advice. Cases where legal and ethical advice conflict suggest that someone getting bioethical advice should also get legal advice so that he or she understands the full ramifications of his or her actions, including the possibility that ethically sound actions may have dire legal consequences. Thus legal pronouncements regarding bioethical issues should not be thought of as dictating the content of bioethical advice; but are, rather, forces independent of bioethics consultation that influence those with the ultimate responsibility for making decisions.

Bioethics committees and consultants are typically not qualified to give legal advice. Only attorneys are licensed to give legal advice, and those who give such advice without a license can be prosecuted for the unauthorized practice of law. One specific aspect of accountability may be a requirement that bioethics consulting services without a licensed attorney must ensure that they do not give legal advice and encourage their clients to seek separate legal counsel. In this fashion, society could be assured that those making bioethical decisions are aware that there are legal as well as ethical factors to be considered.

Closing Comments on Justifying Bioethical Advice

The accountability at issue here does not include being able to present reasons for the advice given that are acceptable to society. In a pluralist society, no one set of ethical reasons is likely to be accepted as the right one, and no one set of ethical conclusions is the only acceptable justification for any given action. The only thing bioethics committees and consultants should be held accountable for is compliance with established procedural rules. The proper consequences of noncompliance depend on how accountability is maintained and, although I advocate in part 4 that some malpractice standards be applied to bioethics consultation, I do not advocate that the content of bioethical advice be regulated to the extent that the content of medical or legal advice is regulated.

In Summary

The accountability used here is a unique concept that should not be confused with other theories of accountability. The primary purpose of accountability is the provision of a uniformly fair and widely applied system for granting and conducting bioethics consultations. Accountability is not a concept based on principles of individual morality but on legal or political fairness. It is not a mechanism for controlling the content of bioethical advice, and it does not require justification for the positions taken by advice givers. It is a mechanism of procedural fairness.

Where We Go From Here

Several fundamental questions must still be answered before we can analyze how bioethics committees and consultants should be held accountable. First, why hold bioethics committees and consultants accountable, and what are the risks and benefits of accountability? This is the topic of the rest of part 1. Second, what models of accountability already exist that we can draw on to establish a prototype for the accountability of bioethics committees and consultants? This will be the topic of parts 2 and 3. And third, once the foregoing questions have been answered, what are some of the specific procedures bioethics committees and consultants should be required to follow? This is the topic of part 4.

CHAPTER TWO

The Accountability of Bioethics Committees and Consultants

The preceding chapter described the general principles of accountability. This chapter argues that those principles should be applied to bioethics committees and consultants.

Background

In the Karen Quinlan case in 1976, the New Jersey Supreme Court suggested that the hospital refer cessation-of-life-support issues to a bioethics committee to help the incompetent patient's doctors and family make their decisions.[1] The use of bioethics committees and consultants has increased dramatically since 1976. Recommendations for the establishment of bioethics committees by the President's Commission for the Study of Ethical Problems in Medicine and Biomedical and Behavioral Research in 1983[2] and the Department of Health and Human Services in 1984[3] precipitated a rapid increase in their use. One state, Maryland, has mandated bioethics committees for all hospitals,[4] and such a mandate has even been considered by the federal government.[5] Finally, the 1992 Joint Commission on Accreditation of Healthcare Organizations' (Joint Commission) requirement that hospitals have a mechanism in place to consider ethical issues arising in the care of patients and to educate caregivers and patients on bioethical issues[6] is likely to further precipitate the growth of bioethics services.

Although it is uncertain what percentage of medical facilities have bioethics consultants, estimates of the percentage of institutions with bioethics committees have grown from between one[7] and sixteen[8] percent to between sixty[9] and ninety[10] percent in the last ten years. The composition of bioethics committees varies, but most committees are dominated by health-care professionals.[11] Participation on bioethics committees is usually voluntary and uncompensated.[12] Some institutions have one full-time committee member or bioethicist to organize committee activities and to keep up with recent developments relevant to those activities.[13] Other institutions do not have a committee, but a bioethics consultant or a team of hospital personnel who act as consultants.[14]

The Goals and Functions of
Bioethics Consultation

Functions performed by bioethics committees and consultants vary widely.[15] Bioethics committees and consultants can provide a forum for airing ethical problems. They can be a resource for persons troubled by the ethical ramifications of decisions made in the medical context. They can help generate hospital policy and educate staff regarding important ethical issues. They can be a sounding board for a variety of ethical perspectives, reflecting the moral viewpoints of not only physicians and academics but also the views of society in general. They can help medical institutions act ethically, that is, they can function as a form of institutional conscience. And perhaps most importantly, bioethics committees and consultants can guide and advise decision makers on considerations they may have overlooked. Through clarifying issues and allowing for open discussion, the committee or consultant can help prevent misunderstandings that could mushroom into full-fledged disputes. Other less common but possible bioethics committee and consultant functions include making macroallocation determinations for medical resources, prognosis confirmation, and reporting staff misconduct to government officials.

All the bioethics committees and consultants I know see their goal as one of giving advice rather than making decisions and as one of education and facilitation rather than dictating moral action. In fact, I have never encountered a bioethics committee or consultant with the last word on what should be done. Even very authoritative committees and consultants claim only to give advisory opinions, leaving the final decision up to patients, their families, friends and surrogates, the medical staff involved in the case, or medical administrators. My desire to provide practical insight into the bioethics consultation debate leads me to accept the advisory role of bioethics committees and consultants as a given rather than arguing that things should be different from how they actually are.

Furthermore, I question the wisdom of suggesting that bioethics committees and consultants should have decision-making authority before there are any mechanisms in place for the provision of even a bare minimum of due process for issues brought to a committee or consultant. In other words, I see the development of mechanisms for assuring accountability as a logical prerequisite to giving bioethics committees and consultants more authority. First, mechanisms should be implemented to help assure that bioethical questions are handled in an appropriate manner. Then, if society becomes more dependent upon bioethics consultation as a means of dispute resolution, bioethics committees and consultants may gain *de facto* decision-making authority or government bodies may consider granting them such authority. The burden of showing why a committee or consultant's advice should not be followed may become very great as society's confidence in bioethics consultation grows. Of course, it is also possible that the public will never gain enough confidence in bioethics consultation to warrant bioethics committees and consultants being granted more authority. In any event, granting bioethics committees and consultants more authority will not endow them with the knowledge and experience so many of them now lack.

Distinguishing Medical from Ethical Concerns

Underlying the functions just described is an important distinction worth exploring. Many patients and their families think medical professionals are "all knowing" when it comes to health care and do not realize that medical and ethical concerns are quite distinct.[16] The health-care professional has the goal and, some would say, obligation to do everything in his or her power to keep patients alive and to aid their recovery.[17] The medical criteria relevant to achieving this goal may not always be clear, but they are dependent upon the medical professional's technical experience, scientific learning, and careful analysis of the patient's physical condition. Ethical decisions are not based on any of these criteria, nor do ethical considerations necessarily suggest the medically indicated decision. Ethical goals vary greatly depending on the theory espoused, but generally, the goal is to achieve what is "right" or "good" for the individual, society, or in general. What is good or right encompasses far more than just physical well-being, although health may be an important factor. In addition to or even instead of considerations of health, ethical deliberations may take into account principles such as quality of life, dignity, integrity, altruism, autonomy, beneficence, nonmaleficience, social welfare, justice, fairness, entitlement, desert, and rights.

Objections to Bioethics Consultation in General

Many objections have been raised against the idea of bioethics committees and consultants. One objection is that they interfere with the patient-physician relationship.[18] This argument stresses that ethical dilemmas are some of the more intimate, delicate problems health-care providers face, and that such problems should be resolved directly with the patient or his or her family, friends, or surrogate.[19] Another objection is that bureaucratic decision making and an effort to arrive at consensus can lead to unacceptable compromises.[20] Also, bioethics committees and consultants are criticized as being inherently prone to a perspective of pragmatic situationism.[21] This is an ethical theory that shies away from dogmatic solutions to ethical dilemmas; problems are solved based on the circumstances of each case.[22] Another common criticism is that bioethics committees and consultants lack either or both the medical and ethical expertise required for sound decision making in the context of ethical dilemmas in medicine.[23] Finally, the most prevalent objection to bioethics committees and consultants is that there is no clear means of assuring their accountability. Some authors suggest that referring decisions to them is used as a means of protecting institutions and physicians from liability.[24] Other authors go so far as to suggest that the possible use of bioethics committees and consultants to diffuse responsibility is a reason to avoid instituting them in the first place.[25] All these objections are in need of response, but for the purposes of this discussion only the accountability issue will be directly addressed.

Arguments Against Holding Bioethics Committees and Consultants Accountable

Here I will discuss some of the major objections to applying formal social mechanisms of accountability to bioethics consultation. What is bioethics and by what criteria can we judge what is sound ethical reasoning? Bioethics is not like medicine where there is a common or authoritative school of learning that makes uniform standards easy to establish. Ethicists have been arguing for millennia about the proper approach to resolving ethical disputes. How then should a bioethics committee or consultant decide which approach to take? Although it is unlikely that a consensus will emerge as to what ethical premises are appropriate, some consensus can be reached on what procedures it would be appropriate for bioethics committees and consultants to follow. Some philosophers argue that the imposition of accountability hinders the functioning of bioethics committees and consultants.[26] They argue that there should be no external check on the functioning of bioethics committees and consultants; the moral consciences of those giving advice is the only form of accountability that will not hinder, to the point of destruction, the functioning of bioethics consultation.[27] These arguments have some merit, but the effect of the problems they raise can be minimized, and the need for accountability far outweighs the possible detrimental effects of assuring accountability.

There are at least three additional aspects of bioethics consultation that create unique accountability problems. First, it is important not to inhibit honest and thorough debate by having committee members or consultants fear lawsuits or other methods of assuring accountability. Second, it is important that bioethics committees and consultants not make decisions, or end up being held accountable for decisions, that properly should be made by health-care personnel, attorneys, patients, or patients' families, proxies, or guardians. In other words, bioethics committees and consultants should not be used as means of avoiding accountability. And finally, when, if at all, should bioethics committees and consultants be held accountable for their advice? Is it really any different when a bioethics committee or consultant gives a doctor or hospital advice than when you or I give a friend advice? Arguably, a bioethics committee or consultant has more influence over a wide range of decisions than you or I, and because of their perceived expertise, their advice is often given more weight than advice coming from other sources. Some possible models for dealing with these accountability problems are explored in parts 2 and 3.

Why We Need to Hold Bioethics Committees and Consultants Accountable

Discussions about accountability by political philosophers can be traced back to arguments justifying the very existence of government. Plato, Aristotle, Hobbes, and Locke, among others, all in one form or another, discuss government as a means of ensuring that its citizens coexist peaceably.[28] Contemporary discussions of accountability are more commonly devoted to questions of the accountability of government to its citizenry.[29] These issues are only very remotely related to the question of accountability I would like to address.

At the heart of my interest in accountability lies a recognition that the difficult questions faced by bioethics committees and consultants do not have easy answers yet ultimately should be handled in the same way--that most bioethical questions are too important to leave up to even the wisest consultants to answer without procedural guidance. Social parameters on how bioethical advice is given are not only desirable but necessary for the well-being of society and the integrity of bioethics. My assertion that there is a need for accountability relies on three arguments: (1) that there is a need for procedural due process, (2) that there is a need for institutional integrity, and (3) that there is a need for professional credibility.

Due Process

Most people are familiar with the phrase "procedural due process" in the context of U.S. constitutional theory. The basic principles behind that theory are the same as those espoused here. Historically, the procedural safeguards of the Fifth and Fourteenth Amendments were intended to create a check on government to prevent the arbitrary infringement of individual freedoms.[30] The prevention of arbitrary loss of freedom is that aspect of procedural due process I would like to stress, but the aspect of that constitutional framework that necessitates checks on government exercise of power is not germane to my thesis. I will argue that the basic principles of procedural fairness are applicable to bioethics consultation because bioethics committees and consultants, albeit unintentionally, could hinder the exercise of individual freedoms cherished by our society.

A Presupposition: The Value of Individual Freedom of Choice

A fundamental presupposition in my argument is that decision-making authority should not be taken away from patients, their families, or surrogates and medical personnel by bioethics committees or consultants. If individual freedom of choice regarding bioethical issues needs to be restricted (and it might need curtailment in some areas), it should be done by government, not by bioethics committees or consultants. The individual exercise of freedom of choice in the medical context, particularly because it is so controversial, is too important a value in our society to allow any curtailment of such freedoms except through the legitimate political processes of our constitutional government.

Procedural Justice

John Rawls, in his book *A Theory of Justice*, uses the example of splitting a cake equally among those who wish to partake to illustrate the working of perfect procedural justice.[31] He points out quite adroitly that procedure is a means for achieving what is agreed upon as a desired end.[32] In the case of the cake, the desired end is equal treatment, and the enabling procedure is to require the one cutting the cake to take the last piece.[33] The constitutional goals of preserving freedom are a little more complicated, but essentially they too involve a desire to give everyone an equal opportunity to enjoy the valued freedoms that constitutionally imposed procedural structures are intended to protect.

The desired end of procedural due process in bioethics consultation is that people are treated fairly in a pluralist society that has, in most instances, not come to any agreement, in the biomedical context, regarding the specifics of what is fair, just, or ethically the right thing to do. Unlike with Rawls's cake, it is not at all clear what the ultimate result to ethical dilemmas should be because these decisions are being made by individuals from a myriad of cultural, religious, and educational backgrounds. The one thing that is true, at least for now, is that in most instances our society has opted to be tolerant of the ethical plurality of its citizens. The desired result, therefore, is not a specific ethical outcome but the protection of individual choice.

I want to emphasize that I am not arguing for perfect procedural justice as described by Rawls.[34] I do not believe that whatever happens according to an agreed-upon procedure is necessarily fair or just. On the contrary, I believe the procedure is necessary specifically because there are so many forms of fairness or justice brought to the bioethics debate. Procedure does not guarantee a correct result, but it does interject a modicum of fairness into how those results are obtained.

Freedom of Choice in the Medical Context

Bioethics consultation developed, in part, due to a perceived need to protect patients' choices. Too frequently patients were not aware of their options or were overwhelmed by authoritative medical figures. Once the movement to help protect patients' freedom of choice gained momentum, those spearheading those efforts realized just how complicated a task they had set for themselves. The task of determining what options a patient had became too great to leave up to just anyone. Soon "experts" emerged in the field of bioethics, and many institutions created task forces or bioethics committees to help solve bioethical problems. Hence we now have a new class of authoritative figures who, very unwittingly at times, may prevent patients, their families, friends, and surrogates, or medical staff from exercising their right to make and act on certain ethical choices.

In such an atmosphere, the best way to help assure that patients, their families, friends, or surrogates, and medical staff are informed, and yet allowed to exercise their freedom to decide bioethical questions for themselves, is to create a system that places checks on how bioethical advice is given. Moreover, the establishment of a procedural structure that is widely applied creates at least a chance that everyone's rights will be protected equally. The fairness that would result from the imposition of such a structure would go a long way toward improving how our society handles bioethical problems by making bioethics consultation a more equitable process.

Institutional Integrity

Those readers familiar with Ronald Dworkin's concept of law as integrity will find much of the argument to come familiar.[35] I will explain Dworkin's position, but the reader must be careful not to try to apply it directly to bioethics consultation. Dworkin is speaking of legal and political integrity, and he does not believe that all institutions must adhere to principles of integrity. I argue that bioethics consultation is an institution where integrity is important for the achievement of accountability. It is also important to note that Dworkin does not discuss integrity as relevant to accountability, and therefore my application of Dworkin's concept of integrity is different from his own. With these caveats having been noted, I proceed to a description of Dworkin's concept of integrity.

Dworkin's Concept of Integrity

For Dworkin, politics is evolutionary rather than axiomatic; it is superimposed upon an existing society that is far from perfect but that is working toward becoming a just state.[36] This approach to the study of law and politics necessitates principles that are not required in the study of static utopias, but must be considered in theorizing about dynamic evolving societies.[37] One such principle is *integrity*.

> [Integrity] requires government to speak with one voice, to act in a principled and coherent manner toward all its citizens, to extend to everyone the substantive standards of justice or fairness it uses for some. . . . [Integrity requires a] state to act on a single, coherent set of principles even when its citizens are divided about what the right principles of justice and fairness really are.[38]

Integrity requires a commitment to consistency for its own sake, and not only procedural consistency but also a degree of consistency in actual decision making.[39] Integrity, in a non-perfect state, must be accepted as an ideal, independent of other principles of fairness and justice, because it can conflict with those principles.[40]

Dworkin argues that this concept of integrity is part of our existing political system.[41] He points out that we would be hard pressed to find someone who would find it acceptable for government to treat similar situations differently on arbitrary grounds.[42] Integrity curbs the range of acceptable methods of assuring fairness.[43] We consider inherently wrong any political compromise that establishes fairness without resolving the underlying moral debate.[44] Dworkin uses the example that we would not accept a proposal to allow abortions only for women born in even years.[45] Another example we would find unacceptable is a system where judges hand out alternating life imprisonment and death sentences to individuals guilty of the same crime. While these compromises are *prima facie* fair, they violate our sense of political integrity--our sense that citizens of a community should share rights and obligations equally.[46] Most people would prefer a law that is consistently applied with which they disagree to the checkerboard-type solutions just described.[47]

Checkerboard decision making is not always bad. Its acceptability depends on the size of the community in question and the issue to be resolved. Although constitutional liberties are nationally enforced, our federalist system allows differences in state laws on many very fundamental issues, for example, the death penalty and abortion. Even smaller realms of decision making exist. Zoning is done at the local level, and certain fundamental questions are left to individual families to decide.

The compromise that allows government to function when people disagree on what is just is *integrity*.[48] Not everyone will agree with every decision, but at least everyone will appreciate that the decisions being made are not arbitrary and that they are to some degree consistent with each other.[49] The state personified lacks integrity if it endorses certain principles to justify some of what it does and then rejects those principles to justify other acts.[50] It is part of our collective political morality to be critical of compromises that allow for arbitrary decision making.[51] Integrity helps preserve equality.[52] Government must pursue a coherent scheme for treating people as equals.[53] Once this notion of integrity is accepted, otherwise puzzling aspects of our political and constitutional structure can be explained.[54] For example, Dworkin discusses the federal system our constitution establishes and how only integrity can explain why it may be constitutionally acceptable for individual states to provide different degrees of protection for individual rights, but why it is not acceptable for a state to make arbitrary distinctions regarding who among its citizens will have their rights protected.[55] A federal system can be fair without requiring that all the states treat their citizens the same as every other state, as long as each state treats its citizens equally. Dworkin then goes on to use integrity as one of the cornerstones for explaining and justifying law as a whole.

My Concept of Integrity

It is important to note that up to this point I have been solely discussing Dworkin's theory. In this section I borrow heavily from Dworkin's ideas but do not apply them directly to bioethics consultation. In reading my explanation of the concept of integrity as it relates to the accountability of bioethics committees and consultants, one should be careful not to confuse Dworkin's own conclusions with my adaptation of his argument.

One reason that I find Dworkin's argument for political integrity so intriguing is that he and I share certain fundamental assumptions about society. We agree that our society is comprised of many individuals with distinct moral perspectives and that our society places great value on respecting those differences.[56] We agree that fairness is a sought-after value in our society.[57] We agree that our society understands impartiality, consistency, and equal treatment as manifestations of fairness.[58] And finally, and perhaps most importantly, we agree on using certain existing structures and principles within society as our starting point for understanding how our society could be improved rather than attempting to theorize in a utopian vacuum.[59] Based on these assumptions, Dworkin argues, as we have seen, that integrity is a political virtue central to our legal system. I, on the other hand, argue--based on these same assumptions--that integrity is an essential reason for holding bioethics committees and consultants accountable.

Not all social institutions must strive to achieve integrity. Dworkin would not argue that religious institutions, for example, need to harmonize all their decisions with accepted social principles the way governments should. Religious organizations appeal to a higher authority than shared social principles. Bioethics consultation, however, unlike religion, is a secular institution that, like government, should be a resource equally available to all those facing bioethical issues independent of their particular moral points of view. Bioethics committees and consultants would be no different from religious counselors if this were not their goal. It is the secular nature of bioethics consultation in a pluralist society that makes integrity an appealing goal and an appealing means of achieving accountability.

The integrity I advocate for bioethics consultation does not require the same form of consistency that Dworkin's concept requires of government. As explained in previous sections, accountability does not require bioethics consultations to result in consistent advice. Quite the contrary, accountability requires only procedural consistency precisely because of the pluralist nature of our society's moral fabric. Governments have the misfortune of having the last word on many difficult moral questions. Bioethics committees and consultants have the luxury of being able to debate bioethics issues without having the burden of fashioning community-wide standards every time they give an opinion. Bioethics committees and consultants can help resolve bioethical problems where government has not made a definitive pronouncement on what should be done, but without having to make the ultimate decision.

Bioethics committees and consultants give advice within the realm of individual choice. They are not decision-making bodies such as legislatures and courts. Their integrity should, at least at this point in history, only be procedural. To demand that bioethics consultations result in consistent advice would be unrealistic and ill conceived. Bioethics committees and consultants would take on a quasi-judicial role, setting precedent before society has come to any consensus as to what is right. As long as our society is sharply divided on what is ethically appropriate conduct, it is best for decision-making authority to rest with patients, their families, or surrogates, and medical staff.

As long as society and government bodies are struggling with bioethical issues and their resolution is left to individual conscience, bioethics committees and consultants should remain free to give whatever advice their deliberations dictate. Unlike courts and legislatures that must act to harmonize their decisions with precedent and the Constitution, there is no authoritative body of decisions or authoritative document that bioethics committees and consultants must apply in making their recommendations. The only harmonization required by accountability is a procedural consistency in how bioethics consultations are handled.

So how does integrity relate to accountability? Integrity is one of the manifestations of fairness that suggests that bioethics consultation should be bound by principles of due process. There is something inherently unfair about how bioethics consultations are presently being conducted. As in the unacceptable checkerboard theory of lawmaking described by Dworkin,[60] bioethics consultations are often conducted in an arbitrary and inconsistent manner. I have not seen any two bioethics consultation services use the same procedures. Many do not even use the same procedure from case to case. Similar cases need not result in similar advice, but the procedures followed in granting and conducting consultations should be consistent.

As consensus grows on bioethical issues, courts and legislatures may choose to make decisions regarding what are and what are not proper choices from a legal standpoint. They may even decide to give bioethics committees and/or consultants some decision-making authority.[61] In either of these situations, government involvement would make integrity necessary to the fullest extent described by Dworkin, but as long as bioethics committees and consultants serve only in an advisory capacity and not as an extension of government's decision-making authority, they should only be held to the weaker standards of procedural integrity I describe.

These principles of institutional integrity are essential to accountability because due process means little if not carried out consistently. Ideally, there should be one primary procedural system followed in all bioethics consultations and that system should be adhered to stringently. Institutional integrity requires a certain degree of equal treatment and respect for individual points of view. It requires equal access to consultation services and a degree of equality of process. It is what makes an otherwise arbitrary set of procedures fair. The procedures established, in and of themselves, may not seem ideal or even fair to everyone, but the fact that they are applied with integrity makes them fair.

Professional Credibility

The profession of bioethics consultation can benefit from accountability. Unlike my previous discussion of how society can benefit from accountability, this section describes what those involved in bioethics consultation will gain by advocating accountability.

At this point I would like to reemphasize that, by concentrating on social accountability, I do not intend to belittle the importance of other types of accountability such as moral accountability. Those involved in bioethics consultation should be concerned with all types of accountability. I only hope that this work can offer some helpful insights regarding aspects of accountability as defined earlier in chapter 1.

A New Field that Lacks Credibility and Guidance

Bioethics consultation lacks credibility because it is a new field. Medical professionals often do not understand the goals or purpose of bioethics consultation. Most patients, their families, or surrogates do not even know that such services exist, let alone that they can avail themselves of them. Part of the confusion is due to the fact that there are as many different notions of what bioethics committees and consultants do as there are bioethics consultation services. Even though most services share the goals of education, facilitating bioethical debate, and dispute resolution, few have established clear procedures for how consultations should be granted and conducted. And, among those programs that have developed procedural standards, none that I know of have uniformly adopted the same standards. Under these circumstances, it is not surprising that hospital personnel, as well as patients and their families, hesitate to avail themselves of bioethics consultation services. They have little idea of what to expect and generally no reason to trust the participants in such programs (for they usually have no evidence of the qualifications of those giving bioethical advice, they may fear their decision-making authority will be usurped; and they may fear the possibility that committee members or consultants will act as whistle blowers), and they have a privacy interest in solving their bioethical problems on their own.

It is also a problem for each bioethics consultation service to have to start from the very beginning in developing its program. There are no generally accepted guidelines for how consultations should be conducted, making it necessary for each new program to survey and evaluate a myriad of existing services. This lack of guidance means it frequently takes years for those developing a consulting service to grasp even the bare mechanics of conducting consultations.

Accountability as a Solution

Due process and integrity can encourage individuals to avail themselves of bioethics consultation services. A formalized structure and procedural safeguards will go a long way toward alleviating individuals' hesitation to use bioethics consultation services. Mechanisms of accountability can serve to make encounters with bioethics services predictable. They can reassure those seeking advice that they will be treated fairly and that their decision-making authority will not be usurped. And, they can vouch for the qualifications of those administering the program.

The mere existence of an outside organization, either public or private, that enforces accountability will bring credibility to consultation services. Individuals who avail themselves of bioethics consultation will feel more secure in the knowledge that a greater authority is supervising consultations. That body may even credential consultation services or provide an avenue for appealing cases where individuals believe their consultation did not meet procedural requirements. Accountability would also minimize the differences between services, thereby making it easier for people to generalize their experiences.

An additional advantage of accountability is the guidance it provides for new bioethics consulting services. The task of starting a new consultation service is simplified through the provision of basic standards. Instead of having each consultant and committee rehash the basic questions of access, training, proceedings, documentation, peer review, appeal procedures, and committee composition, these issues could be settled at the state or national level, thus allowing bioethics committees and consultants to concentrate on the real issues at hand instead of spending most of their time working out administrative formalities.

The Cost of Accountability: A Loss of Professional Independence
The cost of accountability is that those involved in bioethics consultation would lose some freedom in devising their own services; certain procedural aspects of their work would be imposed by an authoritative body. In exchange for this loss of freedom, however, consultation programs would receive guidance and, one hopes, the credibility necessary to encourage individuals to use their services. Furthermore, this loss of freedom can, at least in part, be alleviated by trying to assure that those presently involved in bioethics consultation have considerable input in determining the procedures by which they will be regulated. The degree of input those presently involved in bioethics consultation will have in determining how they are regulated is crucial to part 4's discussion of the relative merits of alternative mechanisms for assuring accountability.

In Summary

The issues being dealt with in bioethics consultation are too important for society not to be concerned about how recommendations are made. There is no social consensus regarding most bioethical issues, and there is no indication that any of the fundamental principles embodied in our law provide clear-cut guidance for the resolution of bioethical questions. Society, however, is not required to let anarchy rule simply because much debate is needed before answers to difficult questions become clear. Certain principles of formal equality, that is, principles of due process, fairness, and consistency, can put some order into the confusion that now reigns. Procedural checks on the process of bioethics consultation can set standards for the airing and handling of disputes. These mechanisms of accountability need not involve government action, but they do need to involve some form of standard-setting authority that can assure consistent and fair application of the procedures it recommends bioethics committees and consultants should follow.

Bioethics committees and consultants also have an interest in assuring their own professional integrity. Mechanisms intended to assure accountability can help build the credibility necessary to encourage use of consulting services. Standards and guidelines also make the actual process of providing bioethics consultation easier.

Accountability should not serve as a mechanism to punish incorrect results because, in many cases, it is unclear which results are correct and which are not.

Where We Go From Here

The most difficult task still lies ahead. Now that we know accountability is a good idea for bioethics committees and consultants, how should we implement the structures needed to assure accountability? Do we have any existing structures that can be adopted as prototypes, or do we need to develop a structure uniquely suited for bioethics consultation? Parts 2 and 3 consider some potential prototypes for assuring the accountability of bioethics committees and consultants.

PART TWO

Some Existing Mechanisms for Assuring Accountability

Introduction to Part Two

Now that we have an idea of why bioethics committees and consultants should be held accountable, it is time to explore some existing structures for assuring accountability. It should be noted that most of the mechanisms described in this part provide accountability in a much broader sense than the accountability central to this book because they regulate content as well as procedure. This fact should not hinder our consideration of these mechanisms as potential prototypes for assuring the accountability of bioethics committees and consultants, but caution should be taken not to carry the analogies further than intended.

This part examines five major types of structures for assuring accountability in the health-care setting. Each of these categories includes a myriad of examples; however, we need only concentrate on a select few for purposes of this discussion. Chapter 3 considers privately imposed, intraprofessional mechanisms such as membership organizations and publication. Chapter 4 considers licensure and medical discipline. Chapter 5 examines government contract controls. Chapter 6 considers judicially enforced accountability, paying particular attention to negligence standards. And chapter 7 focuses on government commissions. Each of these chapters includes a description of the particular mechanisms for assuring accountability and discusses some general advantages and disadvantages of those systems. The appropriateness of applying these mechanisms to bioethics committees and consultants is the subject of part 4.

CHAPTER THREE

Professional Self-Regulation

The three models for accountability discussed here have their origin in the private sector. The first two involve private standard-setting organizations and the third involves peer review through publication.

Standard-Setting Organizations

Private organizations have played a significant role in the development of professional standards. A failure by some organizations to recognize a professional as qualified to practice may result in loss of business or even government denial or revocation of licensure. This discussion will concentrate on two such organizations: those that control accreditation of medical schools and those that control the certification of medical professionals.

Accreditation

This section will discuss the accreditation functions of the American Medical Association (AMA), which is instrumental in developing standards for medical schools.

How Accreditation Works: The AMA's Accreditation of Medical Schools

Accreditation is the process by which an institution is awarded credentials by an organization for having met at least the minimum standards set by that organization. In this case, a private organization has set standards it considers essential for a good medical education.

When it was organized in 1847, the AMA resolved to provide for "the protection of their medical professionals' interests, for the maintenance of their honor and respectability, for the advancement of their knowledge, and the extension of their usefulness."[1] The underlying goal was to protect the trained physician from those who were untrained.[2] One major policy adopted for the achievement of this goal was the development of widely accepted standards for medical education.[3] Thus, educational standards for physicians became one of the AMA's earliest objectives.[4]

Since then, the AMA's many roles have included securing legislative control over professional practices,[5] protecting physicians from federal overregulation,[6] establishing peer review standards, and even hearing disciplinary complaints where local medical societies have shirked their responsibility to deal with such problems.[7]

The AMA of today has eight major functions:

1. Representing doctors on issues that concern them;
2. Providing scientific information through the publication of scientific and educational materials;
3. Providing its members with nonscientific information relevant to the practice of medicine;
4. Keeping statistical data concerning the profession, such as the number of professionals, their geographic locations, and so forth;
5. Setting standards for the accreditation of medical schools, residency training programs, and institutions that offer continuing medical education;
6. Participating in the Joint Commission on Accreditation of Healthcare Organization's (Joint Commission's) efforts to improve the health care provided by medical institutions;
7. Maintaining the AMA's organizational strength by increasing membership, among other things;
8. Providing for the costs of administering the organization.[8]

The educational function upon which this discussion focuses is neither the largest nor the smallest budget item for the AMA.[9]

The AMA is only one of several organizations involved in setting educational standards for the medical profession,[10] but it clearly plays a decisive role. The AMA continuously develops models for schools wishing to upgrade their standards and evaluates schools to see if they meet the AMA's minimum requirements for accreditation.[11] To implement its policies, the AMA, joined by the Association of American Medical Colleges (AAMC), established the Liaison Committee on Medical Education (LCME).[12] The LCME surveys, evaluates, and accredits U.S. medical schools, and thereby controls the quality and content of medical education, the size of classes, and the length of programs.[13]

The AMA is primarily a policy-setting organization, yet it wields considerable influence over entrance into the profession by controlling medical education. In every state a person must be licensed to practice medicine,[14] and in almost every state a person must have attended an AMA-accredited institution (government lists of accredited institutions tend to mirror those of the AMA).[15] More licensure requirements are discussed in chapter 4. With that degree of control over licensure, it is not surprising that medical schools take AMA recommendations for improving their curriculum quite seriously. Milton Friedman writes about how during the Depression the AMA wrote letters to various medical schools admonishing them for taking in more students than they could properly train.[16] Within two years, each school had reduced the number of students it was admitting.[17] Such influence is clearly linked to the fear of losing students if the institution's accreditation is withdrawn.

The Pros and Cons of Accreditation as a Mechanism for Assuring Accountability: Private Interests May Not Coincide with Public Interests

It is hard to argue that setting quality standards can be a bad thing, yet it is possible for accreditation to serve ends that are not in society's best interest. A private organization involved in accreditation may be serving interests other than the maintenance of high standards. For example, the AMA, which is probably the strongest trade union in the country, works to encourage quality medical education as only one of many goals. It has other, perhaps even paramount, goals that can be understood as conflicting with quality control considerations.

The interests of the medical profession, as represented by the AMA, can be considered antithetical to a pure concern for the quality of U.S. health care. Physicians have an interest in limiting their competition and in keeping the cost of health care high so that their profits are greater. Milton Friedman argues that, although this may not be the intention of individual members, the AMA really serves the economic interests of its membership rather than any public interest in quality health care.[18] Under the guise of maintaining high standards, the AMA limits the number of medical students and the number of accredited medical schools, which in turn limits the number of people entering the profession and the number of physicians who need to compete for existing jobs.[19] To support his argument, Friedman gives examples of AMA efforts to limit access to the profession for which no quality control rationales can be found. He discusses the AMA's efforts to require citizenship as a prerequisite for licensure and examinations to be given only in English.[20] Another example is the AMA's hesitancy to accredit foreign medical schools.[21] Examples like these indicate that, at least sometimes, AMA policies are intended to serve economic interests rather than the promotion of high-quality medical services.

Other examples include the AMA's House of Delegates initial failure to approve a report on patients' rights prepared by the AMA Council on Ethical and Judicial Affairs for fear the proposal may attain the standing of a legal standard of care.[22] And, even more recently, the Health Care Financing Administration (HCFA) reported to the House Ways and Means Health Subcommittee that it has started to question the motives and effectiveness of Joint Commission regulation of hospitals.[23] HCFA administrator Gail Wilensky confessed to the committee that HCFA is not certain that Joint Commission accreditation "provides a reasonable assurance that accredited hospitals comply with . . . Medicare standards."[24] It seems it takes the Joint Commission an average of six months after an inspection to notify hospitals with conditional accreditation of deficiencies, and an additional three months or more to determine whether the hospital's corrective measures were sufficient.[25]

On the other hand, some authors point out that such arguments overstate their case. Robert Derbyshire states in his book, *Medical Licensure and Discipline in the United States*, that any binding influence the AMA may have is dependent upon government adoption of its policies.[26] None of the AMA's recommendations have the force of law unless implemented by government.[27] The AMA, through its local membership societies, can refuse or revoke membership, but it cannot restrict or revoke licensure or impose fines.[28] Nor is membership in a medical society ever a prerequisite for licensure, hospital privileges, or certification as a specialist.[29] Thus, the true controller of medical practice is government, which serves many interests other than those of medical professionals, and which has at least the purported goal of looking after the public's general welfare, not just the welfare of physicians.[30]

This debate shows that, if we consider private accreditation as a possible model for the accountability of bioethics committees and consultants, measures should be taken to prevent professional self-interest from predominating social concerns. Furthermore, governments should keep in mind that standards developed by professional organizations may be self-serving; policy makers should consider that possibility carefully before giving professional standards the force of law.

Certification

This section will discuss the certification process as it is carried out by the American Board of Medical Specialties (ABMS), which through its member boards, is instrumental in fashioning the standards individuals must satisfy before they can practice as specialists in a particular area of medicine.

How Certification Works: The ABMS's Certification of Medical Specialists

Certification is the process by which a professional organization recognizes an individual as competent to practice as a member of the profession or in one of its specialties.

The ABMS was organized in 1933 to improve the "quality of health care provided to the public by medical specialists."[31] The ABMS certifies that physicians are qualified specialists through its twenty-three specialty boards,[32] the members of the twenty-three specialty boards are chosen jointly by the ABMS and the AMA.[33] Each member board sets standards that must be met before it allows candidates to sit for its certification examination.[34] Along with educational requirements, the boards require varied degrees of residency training, a specified amount of which must be within the chosen specialty.[35] Once these requirements are met and the comprehensive specialty examination is successfully completed, a physician is board certified within a specific specialty.[36] Several boards also require periodic recertification by examination, and others require participation in continuing education to maintain certification.[37] Most certification boards do not discipline their specialists other than to deny them recertification if requirements are not met or if there is a determination that certification should not have been granted initially.[38] A few boards, however, do allow for possible revocation on more substantive grounds such as suspension of licensure by the state;[39] conviction of a felony or misdemeanor involving moral turpitude;[40] failure to maintain moral, ethical or professional standards;[41] or professional incompetence.[42]

From the physician's perspective, the advantages of specialty certification are primarily economic. Studies show that board-certified specialists[43] can make an average yearly income twenty-six percent greater than noncertified specialists, and that specialists in general have higher incomes than their non-specialized colleagues.[44] Hospital privileges may depend on certification, as may a general public sense of confidence that will lead to a greater number of referrals.[45]

The Pros and Cons of Certification as a Mechanism for Assuring Accountability
Certification Does Not Foreclose Competition the Way Accreditation Historically Has Done

One major advantage of certification is that, unlike accreditation of medical schools, there are no laws in place making certification mandatory. While there are incentives for certification, there is no automatic exclusion of noncertified physicians from the practice of medicine, thus allowing noncertified physicians to compete with certified ones.

Competency Is Not Easy to Measure or Monitor

The major problem with certification is how competency is measured. Even physicians have questioned the value of certification exams.[46] They argue that, while certification appeals to consumers, it really does not say much about a physician's qualifications.[47]

Another problem is that the certification process does little to monitor the continued competency of physicians. Perhaps organizations involved in certification should take a more active role in reevaluating their specialists. The efforts made by some certification boards to require recertification or expand the conditions under which they are willing to consider revocation of certification are a step in the right direction, but other efforts should also be made to monitor whether a broader range of professional standards is being met. Certifying organizations could conduct occasional on-site reviews of physician practices, or, perhaps more realistically, certifying organizations could depend on the evaluation of other private and governmental organizations to make determinations of whether or not a physician has dropped below the organization's minimum standards. More extensive involvement in the monitoring of professional competency would require most certifying organizations to expand their standards to include considerations other than the satisfaction of educational requirements.

Publication

Scientists, academics, and others have traditionally published their work to make it available for consideration by their peers, and to receive comments that might help further develop their ideas. For example, from its inception, the AMA has had the goal of advancing the knowledge of its members.[48] Working to improve medical education is one method pursued by the AMA to achieve this goal; another is the dissemination of information.[49] In recent years, the AMA has spent the major part of its budget on providing information to physicians, government, and the general public.[50] To that end, the AMA publishes ten journals and a multitude of other scientific and educational materials.[51]

How Publication Works

Publication can serve numerous ends. It is a means of reaching a large audience. It is one of the best ways to disseminate information rapidly and accurately. For someone who may want to have a new idea tried or accepted by a large number of people or by his or her peers, publication is necessary so that others can learn of the idea. Publication in professional journals allows for intellectual discourse with one's colleagues. The value of such discourse is the transmittal of knowledge, the consideration and evaluation of ideas by a large peer group, and the potential for constructive criticism.

Publication can also function as a mechanism of accountability. If the activities of a professional or professional group (for example, minutes or case summaries) are published and reviewed on a regular basis, those activities could be subject to peer approval or disapproval. Such peer pressure can be very effective in curtailing unacceptable practices. For example, some have contended that failure to agree with AMA policy can result in pressures ranging from social ostracism to professional boycott.[52]

The Pros and Cons of Publication as a Mechanism for Assuring Accountability

There are two issues that need to be considered in discussing the value of publication as a mechanism for assuring accountability: (1) the potential role of publication in developing the specific procedures of accountability, and (2) the potential role of publication as a mechanism for implementing these procedures.

The Specific Procedures of Accountability

The only argument for using publication as a method of developing the actual procedures of accountability is that publication allows a very large number of people to be involved in the refinement of ideas. This argument is essentially the one made by John Stuart Mill in his work *On Liberty*[53] for what has come to be known as the "free marketplace of ideas." Mill argues that exposing an idea to a wide audience allows criticisms that will aid in the refinement of those ideas, bringing them closer to the truth and closer to broad acceptance.[54] The more that information is disseminated, the more knowledgeable individuals become, and the more equipped they are to make enlightened decisions.[55] Unfortunately, as even Mill realized, access to truth is more complicated than merely assuring open debate.

The Access Fallacy

One major problem with a free marketplace of ideas is access to the medium. Where will ideas be published? Who will be reached? And who will bother to respond? The answers to these questions already severely limit those with access to the debate. Which of the myriad of bioethics journals will take up the issue of consultation procedures? How can any human being, even one with the utmost interest in the subject, stay abreast of everything written on the subject? How can we guarantee that all those who have something worthwhile to say will try to publish or be published if they try? Wealth, education, social and academic standing, writing ability, and numerous other factors independent of the value of the ideas being presented influence who writes, who is published, and who reads what is published.

The Failed Pursuit of Truth

There is also the question of whether the broad acceptance of an idea in any way indicates its truth. Popular acceptance only indicates that the majority has been convinced of a certain point of view, not that the majority is correct. I would contend that one should rather take the advice of one Socrates than the advice of one hundred not so wise. Thus the advice of a few experts who have seriously considered the problem would be preferable to the conclusions reached by a more open debate such as publication. On the other hand, open debate may be a crucial precursor to expert decision making because it aids in the dissemination of information.

The High Cost of Consensus

Finally, publication, even if the consensus desired is only among the members of a very select audience, is a time-consuming method of conducting a debate. For publication to serve as a mechanism for developing procedures for holding bioethics committees and consultants accountable, some form of consensus would have to be reached. Many issues have been debated without resolution for decades or centuries. Frequently, debate even continues after government or some other authoritative body has taken action to implement its preferred perspective. Some concerns simply are too pressing to allow for the amount of time it takes to arrive at a consensus through publication. Nevertheless, conducting a debate in print can make valuable contributions for the consideration of those more directly involved in devising procedures for assuring the accountability of bioethics committees and consultants.

Enforcing Accountability
How Publication Can Be Used to Enforce Accountability
    Publication fares better as a mechanism for assuring accountability than it does as a mechanism for developing a specific process for assuring accountability. Once a given process has been chosen, even if only by members of a private organization, publication could help assure that mandated procedures are actually followed by providing an avenue for public scrutiny or peer review.

How Publication Might Encourage Conservatism
    As appealing as publication is as a mechanism for assuring accountability, it is not without problems. People who know their actions are open to public scrutiny may become overly cautious. A fear of criticism may cause people to hesitate to argue extreme positions or prevent them from criticizing each other for fear of embarrassing their colleagues or of being criticized in return.
    In response it could be argued that, while it is understandable why someone might not defend a position he or she does not believe in for fear of being misunderstood as advocating that position, most people are probably not embarrassed to advocate their own heartfelt ideas. If people have misgivings about a position they are about to take, perhaps there is no harm in their reconsidering before expressing their thoughts.

How Publication Could Compromise Patient Confidentiality
    Regardless of what approach is taken to publication, if it is employed as a mechanism for assuring accountability in the medical context, patient confidentiality could be compromised. The degree to which the facts of a case would need to be disclosed in order for accountability to be assured would depend on the specific procedures implemented to assure such accountability. Certainly, a patient's name would not need to be disclosed, but some have argued that the identification of a patient by initials is essential for cross reference to other reports about the same patient.[56] Others have argued that identification of a patient can happen even without the use of the patient's name or initials simply because of the details given regarding the facts of the case. The patient or his or

her family could suffer considerable distress or embarrassment if a patient is identified as the subject of an article.[57]

Accountability may be achievable without compromising confidentiality because of the type of review involved. For scientific or medical analysis of a case, a detailed description of a patient's medical history and condition is necessary, but fewer details are required to analyze whether proper procedures were followed.

The Feasibility of Publication

It is also questionable whether publication is always feasible. Publication is costly and time consuming. Particularly if the publication of minutes or case summaries is required, the mere volume of material may make careful scrutiny impossible. In response, it can be argued that accountability is worth the time and expense publication requires. As a possible compromise, however, publication could be limited to specific reviewers, or the reports required could be very sketchy and reviewers could be allowed to request more details on a spot-check basis.

Incidental Benefits

In addition to functioning as a mechanism for assuring accountability, the publication of case reports or meeting minutes could have other benefits. Such publication allows others to learn by example. It allows difficult issues to be aired. It gives readers an opportunity to consider problems before they have to face them themselves. And, it provides others involved in bioethics consultation new and different insights into how certain types of cases can be handled and resolved.

In Summary

The assurance of accountability through self-regulation is not new to the medical setting. Mechanisms such as accreditation, certification, and publication have been effective, albeit not perfect, means of regulating professional conduct for centuries. The primary disadvantage of the three mechanisms discussed in this chapter is also their primary advantage: they are mechanisms that are self-imposed by a profession. The clear advantage of such mechanisms is that they are implemented and enforced by those most qualified to judge professional competence--namely, professionals themselves. On the other hand, self-regulation may promote self-interest at the expense of public interests and result in an inefficient system for providing accountability.

Where We Go From Here

Ironically, the problems of self-regulation extend beyond the private sector into the public realm of government regulation. In the next chapter we will see that licensure and medical disciplinary measures are plagued by many of the same problems as professional self-regulation because governments have relied heavily on the private sector for guidance on how medical professionals should be regulated.

CHAPTER FOUR

Licensure and Professional Discipline

Questions of professional self-regulation and government regulation of licensure and professional discipline are more closely related than one might think. Licensure requirements are usually based on standards developed by the profession and medical disciplinary bodies. And, although technically part of state governments, medical disciplinary bodies are almost exclusively made up of medical professionals.

The mechanisms of accountability discussed in this chapter, unlike those in chapter 3, are public and, unlike those in chapter 5, originate at the state rather than the federal level. This chapter concentrates on the licensure and disciplining of medical professionals.

Licensure

The federal government's definition of *licensure* is as follows:

[Licensure is] the process by which an agency of government grants permission to persons to engage in a given profession or occupation by certifying that those licensed have obtained a minimal degree of competency to insure that the public health, safety and welfare will be reasonably well protected.[1]

How Licensure Works

Some form of medical licensure has been in existence in the United States for over 150 years.[2] The goal of licensure is to limit entry into the profession to those who have met minimal requirements. Licensure requirements then serve as the standard applied in making medical disciplinary decisions.

Nowhere in this country can a physician legally practice without a license. Every state's requirements are unique, but there are some fundamental similarities. For example, most states rely on either the Federation of State Medical Board Licensing Examination (FLEX) or the National Board of Medical Examiners Examination (NBME) for a determination of a basic competency to practice medicine. Other common requirements include educational requirements (that is, applicants must have attended an accredited medical school), post-graduate training, and a demonstration of moral fitness to practice medicine.

Most states have one agency, called the "medical board," that licenses medical professionals. Medical boards are usually independent state agencies, although they may be part of other health, consumer, or business-related departments. The licensing function performed by medical boards includes the examination of an applicant's credentials for academic and moral fitness. Medical boards administer the state's licensing exam (usually the FLEX or NBME), monitor medical schools, and promulgate standard-setting regulations.

The composition of medical boards varies considerably from state to state. Tennessee, for example, has two boards involved in medical licensing.[3] One has five physician or surgeon members; the other has three members from any of the healing arts professions.[4] New York has a licensing board of at least twenty physicians.[5] Most states have medical boards dominated by medical professionals. If states allow lay members at all, they usually allow only one or two token public representatives.[6]

In many states medical boards are part-time agencies whose members are only paid a small per-diem allowance. Thus, professionals who serve on such boards see their membership as primarily honorific and spend most of their time pursuing more lucrative endeavors.[7]

The appointment of medical board members may even be controlled by local medical societies. For example, in Maryland, until recently, the State Medical and Chirurgical Faculty elected the entire licensing board.[8] In other states, like Alabama, the local medical society actually serves as the licensing board.[9] And, in most other states, the local society submits to government agencies a list of candidates from which appointments are generally made.[10] Thus, in most states, medical societies either directly or indirectly control who serves on medical boards.

The Pros and Cons of Licensure as a Mechanism for Assuring Accountability

Government Action

Governments, at least in theory, serve the public interest, not special interests such as those represented by the AMA. Governments are also ultimately responsible to the public through a democratic system of government. Private organizations are only accountable to their members. Thus licensure provides for the possibility of non-self-interested control of professional conduct.

Furthermore, without mandatory government licensure, there would be no justification for government disciplinary measures. Medical societies can banish someone from their ranks, causing bad publicity and a loss of business, but their actions cannot prevent a physician from practicing medicine. Only government agencies have the authority and the power to actually prevent incompetent physicians from practicing medicine. Thus government licensure is required if disciplinary action is going to be effective.

Government Inaction

Unfortunately, few states have taken their role as protectors of the public against professional incompetence as seriously as one might like. Too often the standards adopted for licensure are directly dictated by the very profession being regulated. Chapter 3 discussed the AMA's influence on licensure requirements, and we have seen in this section how licensing boards are dominated by medical professionals. In many instances, state governments merely take the standards provided by the profession and give them the force of law.

Reliance on the profession for guidance is understandable because of the degree of expertise at issue, but efforts should be made to weed out policies motivated by professional self-interest when establishing licensure requirements. Physician contributions certainly are helpful, but they need not be the only, or primary, instigators of licensure policies. More nonphysicians need to be involved in setting licensure standards.

Professional Discipline

How Medical Discipline Works

Medical disciplinary action is action taken by government agencies to discourage unprofessional conduct among medical professionals after they have been licensed to practice medicine. Discipline is a logical extension of a government's licensing authority. While licensing tries to limit entry into practice to those who have proven at least a minimal degree of competency, discipline is a mechanism for responding to deviations from good practice. The standards applied for determining licensure are also used for deciding where disciplinary action is required.

Each state has a unique disciplinary system. In most states, the medical boards responsible for licensing are also responsible for taking disciplinary action. A description of those boards was given in the last section, so it will not be repeated here. In those states where disciplinary and licensing functions are separate, the disciplinary function is carried out by an independent board, or an agency with the power to discipline professionals in general or some other government body. However, even in states with independent disciplinary functions, the disciplining of physicians is to a large extent controlled by physicians and their medical societies.

Generally, medical practice laws enumerate the grounds for disciplinary action. The types of conduct for which disciplinary action can be taken usually fall into one of the following categories:[11]

1. Unprofessional conduct;
2. Conviction of a felony or offense involving moral turpitude;
3. Substance abuse or drug dealing;
4. Violation of abortion laws;
5. Fraud in licensure application or examination or other types of fraud;
6. Mental, physical, or other inability to practice medicine safely;
7. Discipline or revocation of license in another state;
8. Breaching patient confidentiality or revealing other privileged information;
9. Malpractice;
10. Fee-splitting;
11. Violation of the Controlled Substances Act;
12. Violation of the Medical Practice Act;
13. Immorality;
14. Other less serious violations of licensure requirements, such as misuse of the title MD or failure to display one's license or pay one's licensing fee.

In accordance with medical practice laws, medical boards dismiss, mediate, settle, or pursue legal action in response to complaints received. Medical boards usually have the authority to subpoena witnesses and determine penalties, but they do not always have an adequate number of investigators, hearing officers, or attorneys to process all the complaints received.[12] In some states, the medical board makes decisions that can be appealed in the courts, and in others the courts make the initial decision, which the board then reviews and can modify.[13]

The Pros and Cons of Medical Discipline as a Mechanism for Assuring Accountability

Government Intervention

Government involvement, as was pointed out in our discussion of licensure, in principle provides a structure free from the private interests likely to dominate private organizations involved in professional self-regulation. Moreover, government involvement is necessary to provide disciplinary bodies with the legal authority to impose and enforce penalties when necessary.

The major disadvantage of government involvement is that, in the existing system of licensure and medical discipline, too much reliance is placed on the judgment of medical professionals regarding the standards they should be required to meet. Earlier sections discussed how medical boards are dominated by physicians with perhaps only token lay representation. The compassion that physician-dominated boards feel for their erring colleagues may result in disciplinary actions too lenient to truly protect the public interest.

Another disadvantage to any form of government regulation, particularly if it is going to be carried out efficiently, is that public funds are required. When government becomes involved, taxpayers must pay for the development and maintenance of whatever system is established for the assurance of accountability. When professionals regulate themselves, they, not the public at large, are primarily responsible for bearing the cost of assuring accountability.

The Effect of Government Intervention on the Profession

One general argument against government involvement that underlies most arguments in favor of professional self-regulation stems from the definition of *profession*. Sociologist Elliot Freidson argues that professionals claim to possess such a high degree of skill that persons who are not members of the profession do not have the requisite knowledge required to evaluate professional conduct.[14] (This is the same type of rationale that makes medical experts so indispensable in malpractice suits.) Others add that to allow nonprofessionals to regulate professionals damages professional integrity and entangles professional conduct regulation unnecessarily in government bureaucracy.[15] The obvious retort to this argument is that professional self-regulation is wonderful as long as it in fact works. As we will see in the next section, leaving physicians to discipline themselves has not always proved effective.

Is the Existing System of Medical Discipline Effective?

The disciplinary record of medical boards is hardly exemplary, even though the number of physicians unfit to practice is potentially very great. Robert Derbyshire, in his book *Medical Licensing and Discipline in the United States,* estimates that one in twenty physicians is a "problem doctor": is incompetent or dishonest, has committed a felony, or has a substance abuse problem.[16] Analysis of statistics available from the Federation of State Medical Boards and the AMA reveal that in 1985, on the average, only 3.8 out of one thousand physicians were disciplined and only 0.7 out of one thousand had their licenses revoked.[17] With so few physicians being disciplined, even if Derbyshire's estimates are grossly exaggerated, there still are many problem doctors who have gone undisciplined under the existing system.[18]

In Summary

Government involvement in the regulation of medical professionals through licensing and disciplinary boards, in theory, is necessary to help assure that professionals do not further their own interests at public expense. Unfortunately, the existing licensing and disciplinary system is dominated by the very interests government intervention should control. Such failings, however, are not incurable. The improvement of licensing and medical disciplinary procedures could begin by increasing lay representation, increasing board investigative powers, and providing better funding for board members and staff, so that boards can investigate more thoroughly and respond more effectively to complaints received.

Where We Go From Here

Now that we have examined professional self-regulation and state regulation dominated by professional interests, it is time to turn to a government-administered type of control that is far more independent of professional influences. Chapter 5 discusses how government contracts can be used to assure accountability in the medical setting.

CHAPTER FIVE

Government Contracting

There are a myriad of examples of government regulatory systems. It would take tomes to describe those in the health-care area alone. This book discusses several forms of government regulation. Licensure and medical discipline were considered in the last chapter. Court-enforced accountability and government commissions are looked at in the next two chapters. Part 3 explores government involvement in the regulation of Institutional Review Boards (IRB) and peer review committees. And this chapter will discuss government contracts. The particular government contract model considered here is the system governing Peer Review Organizations (PRO). PROs are mechanisms external to the health-care delivery system that consist of private physician organizations that contract with the government to provide quality-assurance review. These organizations are of interest because, although they are private, they were created in accordance with a federal mandate and are strictly controlled by the terms of their government contracts.

How Peer Review Organizations Work

From its inception, utilization review by medical institutions was part of the Medicare program.[1] Unfortunately, this review was not performed to the satisfaction of the federal government, so in 1972 the Professional Standards Review Organization (PSRO) law established 203 physician groups to review care rendered to Medicare and Medicaid patients.[2] PSROs were mandated to determine the following:

1. Whether the services paid for by the federal government were reasonable and necessary;
2. Whether professional standards for quality service were being met;
3. Whether the services being rendered could be provided more economically by another type of medical facility, for example skilled nursing facilities.[3]

In 1982 the PSRO law was repealed due to its failure to show clear positive financial impact,[4] and in its place the Quality Control Peer Review Organization (PRO) statute was enacted.[5]

The PRO law replaced the local PSRO groups with statewide organizations and provided for negotiated numerical contract objectives for evaluating whether the PRO was performing as required.[6] In addition to the earlier goals set by PSRO laws, PROs were also to review these points:

1.   Whether complete, adequate, and quality care was being provided;
2.   Whether the diagnostic and procedural information submitted by hospitals was a valid basis for determining the diagnosis-related groups (DRG) upon which federal reimbursement was based;
3.   Whether unusually long stays or high costs for services were warranted in particular cases;
4.   Whether a medical institution was guilty of misconduct in admission or discharge procedures or other practices with respect to beneficiaries or the billing of beneficiaries, such as unnecessary admissions or fallacious discharge information.[7]

As under the PSRO system, a PRO determination of misconduct could result in denial of federal payment for services, fines, or even exclusion from Medicare.[8] Today PROs function more as quality-assurance organizations than as utilization-review organizations, although all of these objectives still remain in place.[9]

Some substantive regulations for how the PRO process should work were published by the Department of Health and Human Services (DHHS) in 1985,[10] but an interim manual also published by DHHS and only available from DHHS or the National Technical Information Service is the primary source of PRO requirements. Newer, more extensive regulations are available only in proposed form.[11]

The Pros and Cons of Government Contracting as a Mechanism for Assuring Accountability

It is too early to evaluate whether PROs are meeting their newest goal of assuring quality medical care. Nevertheless, there seem to be some general benefits to the government contract model of assuring accountability, and only a few disadvantages, if any.

Funding

The primary disadvantage of the PRO system is that it is totally funded at government expense. And, as was mentioned in my earlier discussion of medical licensure and discipline, it is not easy to gain support for government funding, particularly if private alternatives exist. The major reason the PRO system was funded was because of its potential for cutting Medicare and Medicaid costs.

Contractual Constraints

PROs are private organizations, but they were formed to provide a statutorily mandated service. The federal government has total control over the goals and functioning of PROs. Thus, unlike the private membership organizations and the state medical boards dominated by the members of those organizations discussed in chapters 3 and 4, there is little room for PROs to serve professional interests at the expense of public interests. If a PRO does not satisfy the specific terms of its contract to the government's satisfaction, the government has the option of not renewing its contract, and the PRO will go out of business. PROs are totally dependent on the government for their continued existence. They cannot toy with serving interests other than those contractually stipulated because to do so can mean financial ruin.

Competition

Not only do PROs have to worry about meeting their contractual obligations, but they have to compete for their contracts. In order to compete, PROs must devise efficient and inexpensive ways of providing government the services it desires. For example, in the 1988 contracting cycle, the Illinois PRO promised to reduce the number of admissions for eleven specific DRGs by more than 7,000 unnecessary admissions by performing a 100 percent retrospective review of all hospitals.[12] Such a thorough evaluation of services would not be likely under the private or public forms of regulation discussed in earlier chapters.

One potential drawback of such competition is that the intense desire to receive such a contract can lead to the bribing of government officials, payoffs, and the unfair evaluation of bids. While the possibility of such corruption is very real, it is not necessarily the system that is to be faulted, but those implementing the system. Efforts should be made to curb government corruption, but the specifics of how such a goal can be achieved are beyond the scope of this discussion.

Professional Know-How

One very major advantage of the government contracting model over some other possible forms of government regulation is the degree to which professionals can be relied upon to do a fair assessment of their peers' work. Because of the competitive contractual nature of PROs, their member physicians cannot afford to be lenient or overly sympathetic to colleague physicians who are not meeting required quality control standards. Unlike physicians involved in private membership organizations or even medical boards, the livelihoods of PRO physicians are directly linked to their ability to be critical of their colleagues' performance.

In Summary

Government contracts in the area of health care may be the form of government regulation that can best draw on the advantages of professional self-regulation without incorporating all of its disadvantages. However, as advantageous as such a system may seem, it carries a considerable price tag when applied in an area where government is not already bearing the expense of providing for the services being rendered.

Where We Go From Here

The next two chapters deal with other types of government mechanisms for assuring accountability. Chapter 6 discusses the courts, which can impose the most severe penalties for misconduct of any government body involved in assuring accountability. Chapter 7 discusses government commissions that, in and of themselves, have no enforcement power and are totally dependent upon other mechanisms of accountability for the weight their guidance carries.

CHAPTER SIX

Judicial Remedies

Probably the most common and, in many ways, the most effective means of ensuring accountability is by threat of judicial intervention. Professionals and those with whom they work are susceptible to a myriad of different legal claims for improper conduct. This chapter will concentrate on the application of negligence principles as a possible mechanism for assuring accountability but will also briefly discuss some other forms of liability.

How Court-Enforced Accountability Works

Courts are adjudicative bodies whose decisions have the force of law. Unlike private organizations that may threaten loss of membership and bad publicity, or medical boards that can restrict a physician's ability to practice or impose fines, courts have a far greater and more far-reaching authority.

Most people, and certainly most medical professionals, understand all too well the dangers of court intervention. For all concerned, defendants and plaintiffs alike, legal actions are time consuming, emotionally trying, and expensive. For medical professionals who are defendants, even if they win, their reputations and ability to attract patients may be severely hampered. And, if they lose, they can suffer astronomical civil or even criminal penalties.

This section discusses some of the legal theories that can lead to such liability, with an emphasis on tort[1] claims for negligence because those are the types of claims most likely to be raised against bioethics committees and consultants.

Negligence

Negligence is a kind of conduct from which liability will follow. A cause of action for negligence has four necessary elements:

1. A duty or obligation, recognized by law, to act in accordance with a specific standard of conduct necessary to protect others from unreasonable risks;
2. A failure to comply with the duty expressed in 1, above;

3. A sufficient causal connection between that failure and a resulting injury;
4. An actual loss or damage due to the injury mentioned in 3, above.[2]

For the ordinary person, the duty recognized by law is to exercise the degree of care that an ordinarily prudent person would exercise under the same or similar circumstances.[3]

Malpractice

A malpractice action requires the same four basic elements required for an ordinary negligence claim, but the care legally expected of a professional in the exercise of his or her profession is different from the care expected of a lay person. The duty owed by a person of superior knowledge or skill is to use reasonable care in light of those special abilities.[4] Thus, a physician could be negligent in cases where an ordinary person would not, and a medical specialist could be negligent where an ordinary physician would not, because of their relative abilities.

In addition to acting reasonably, given their special abilities, professionals are negligent if they lack the special skill or knowledge expected of the average, prudent member of their profession.[5] This standard usually manifests itself as an obligation to comply with the minimum standards of the profession.[6]

Physician Consultants

There must be a patient-physician relationship before the duty element of a negligence claim against any physician can be met. This is also true of physician consultants. For a consultant to have a duty of care for a particular patient, a relationship must have been initiated, with that patient's care in mind.[7] That relationship need not be directly with the patient; it can be with the patient's treating physician, but an acknowledgment of the relationship by the consultant is required before he or she can be considered as having a duty to the patient.[8] Informal discussion of a patient with another physician does not suffice.[9] But examination of the patient and his or her records, making a recommendation to the treating physician, and charging a consultation fee are evidence that a patient-physician relationship exists and, consequently, a duty to provide reasonable care.[10]

Once the consultant's duty toward a patient is established, the other three elements of a negligence claim must be satisfied to the same extent they would for any other physician with the consultant's specific skills or knowledge.[11]

Clergy

Although physician liability for malpractice is the most developed area of malpractice law, the liability of religious counselors provides a closer analogy to bioethics consultants because both give advice that can be understood as ethical advice. Unfortunately, as with bioethics committees and consultants themselves, the law in this area is just beginning to develop, and it is uncertain if such liability exists. In one unreported case (settled and sealed by the court for privacy reasons), the court recognized a separate and distinct claim for clergy malpractice.[12] However, no reported opinions have recognized such a cause of action and only two reported cases even discuss the possibility of clergy malpractice. In the recently decided case of *Nally v. Grace Community Church of the Valley*,[13] the California Supreme Court rejected the possibility of clergy malpractice by holding that a clergy does not have a duty to refer a potentially suicidal person to mental health professionals. And, in *Lund v. Caple*,[14] the Washington Supreme Court denied any malpractice claims for a clergyman's sexual "misconduct."[15] Clergy malpractice, however, is an important area of law to watch as a possible predictor for whether bioethics committees and consultants could be held liable for their advice.

Fiduciary Duties

Another attenuated but somewhat relevant analogy is the liability of corporate directors, attorneys, accountants, brokers, trustees, and others who give professional advice. For simplicity, this discussion will focus on the liability of corporate directors, but it cannot be assumed that what is said here is equally applicable to other professionals. Although the fiduciary principles underlying the liability for professional advice are similar, each profession has its unique obligations.[16]

Directors are subject to the ordinary prudent-person standard of care, but that standard is tempered by a fiduciary duty to the corporation (and its shareholders).[17] Directors are required to act honestly, in good faith, and to deal fairly with the corporation's best interest at heart.[18] Courts often express these duties in lofty terms. One court stated that directors owe "loyalty and allegiance to the corporation--a loyalty that is undivided and an allegiance that is influenced in action by no consideration other than the welfare of the corporation."[19] Some courts even require directors to prevent their own passive negligence, that is, impose a duty on directors to prevent the illegal conduct of others.[20] To hold directors liable for their advice, plaintiffs (usually disgruntled shareholders) must show a breach of duty and prove that the breach was the proximate cause of their loss.[21] However, where directors act within their granted authority (*intra vires*), act with a reasonable basis for their decision (due care), and do not breach their fiduciary duties (act honestly and in good faith with their corporation's best interests in mind), they are protected by the "business judgment" rule.[22] Under this defense, directors are given considerable discretion, even if their decisions end up being detrimental to the corporation, as long as their actions meet the three conditions just described.[23]

Some Other Theories of Liability

This section is not so much included to demonstrate how legal liability can function as a mechanism for assuring accountability as to list some other legal theories that potentially could be used against bioethics committees and consultants. Keep these possibilities in mind when part 4 discusses limiting bioethics committee and consultant liability.

1. Intentional infliction of emotional distress. This tort requires that an actor's extreme and outrageous, intentional, or reckless conduct causes severe emotional distress in another.[24]
2. Defamation. This tort requires a communication to at least one third party that tends to injure reputation in the commonly understood sense of the word: that what was communicated tended to injure esteem, respect, good will, confidence, or excite derogatory or unpleasant feelings or opinions toward the plaintiff.[25]
3. Civil rights violations. Civil rights are any individual or minority rights the government protects against its own actions or those of private individuals. Civil rights are protected by federal and state constitutions, and by legislation passed by Congress or the states.[26] Cases are generally brought for the unjustifiable consideration of race, age, religion, sex, marital status, handicap, or other unacceptable forms of discrimination.[27]
4. Criminal prosecution. Any time a crime is committed, others may potentially be involved as conspirators.

The Pros and Cons of Court-Enforced Accountability

It would take volumes to even mention all the possible advantages and disadvantages of our judicial system. This section will discuss only those concerns that will be most relevant to our later discussion of the accountability of bioethics committees and consultants.

Public Versus Private

The court system is a branch of government removed enough from political pressure that, unlike state regulatory bodies, it does not suffer from the problems of self-interest that potentially permeate the private sector. The judiciary is, in principle, unbiased, and the judicial system's procedural safeguards are intended to assure fair consideration of relevant issues.

Also, unlike decisions made by private organizations, court decisions have the force of law. The threat of litigation and the possible penalties associated with a finding of guilt are undoubtedly a stronger deterrent than loss of membership in a private organization or even the loss of licensure.

The public nature and strong deterrent power of the courts, however, also pose potential problems not likely to surface when private organizations consider disciplining their members. Courts are public institutions, and all the accusations filed against a defendant are generally of public record. Private organizations may keep the fact that they are investigating possible misconduct a secret, sparing those that are found innocent the humiliation and potential loss of business that can result from even an unfounded accusation. The courts cannot protect defendants from the consequences of being accused of wrongdoing even if they are proved innocent.

Fear of Litigation

The fact that mere litigation of a case, whether one is justly accused or not, carries with it so many penalties (cost, humiliation, time, emotional stress, loss of business, and more) makes it a threat that is independent of the threat of being found guilty. The fear of litigation itself may be so great that it overtakes the fear of doing wrong and actually, on occasion, encourages misconduct. A commonly employed example is that of a physician who pursues aggressive treatment on a dying patient, contrary to the patient's wishes, for fear of being accused of not having done everything possible to save the patient's life.

A fear of litigation may also discourage people from becoming involved in activities where the risk of litigation is high even if the risk of actually being found culpable for misconduct is low. For example, an excellent physician may stop providing certain services because of a high risk that he or she will be accused of malpractice or because the malpractice insurance premiums for such services are prohibitively expensive.

In Summary

Judicial intervention is a powerful tool for assuring accountability that is free, for the most part, of control by private interests. On the other hand, the public nature of trials makes the mere threat of litigation, rather than the threat of being found guilty, a great disadvantage. It can discourage innovative practices and prevent people from entering or staying in a field for fear of being falsely accused of wrongdoing.

Where We Go From Here

Now that we have considered private self-regulation, administrative regulation, and judicial remedies, there is only one more type of mechanism for assuring accountability worthy of our attention: government commissions. These quasi-governmental bodies are important because of their potential role as standard-setting organizations.

CHAPTER SEVEN

Government Commissions

Government commissions are very weak mechanisms for assuring accountability. Strictly speaking, they only *influence* other mechanisms for assuring accountability, rather than being such mechanisms themselves. Despite this limitation, government commissions are worth exploring because their influence on how mechanisms of accountability develop could potentially be very great.

There have been hundreds, if not thousands, of government commissions on the state and federal level. Each commission or consultative body has its own unique structure, mandate, time-frame, and influence, making it extremely difficult to generalize and even more difficult to pull out just one or two examples of typical commissions. Thus, this chapter will discuss several well-known federal commissions to illustrate a variety of points rather than describe one or two in detail.

How Government Commissions Work

Having pointed out that it is difficult to generalize, I will begin by trying to do just that. Government commissions are standing bodies or *ad hoc* groups headed by a collegial body of commissioners and, for our purposes, are generally temporary and oriented toward solving a particular social problem or issue.[1] They are usually formed by legislative mandate, although they can have their origins in any branch of government. They report to some government body, usually the legislature, the president, or a particular government agency, on an existing or expected social problem.

Government commissions may be mandated to collect data, to study and evaluate potential problems, and/or to make actual policy recommendations, but they usually serve one of six functions:

1. They can legitimize government actions by giving an apparently impartial endorsement of the action;

2. They can delay the need for government resolution of a controversial issue;
3. They can identify duplications in government efforts and foster cooperation among government agencies or programs;
4. They can form a representational function if the commissioners hold diverse viewpoints;
5. They can perform a fact-finding function by conducting research;
6. They can educate the public and/or government, and build public support for policy changes.[2]

Commission members are appointed by the legislature or whichever government body the commission is to advise. Usually members are picked for their ability to make a valuable contribution to the commission's work, but such considerations are often coupled with less relevant political considerations such as party affiliation and administrative or industry contacts.

The influence that commissions have depends on a variety of factors. For example, when Congress authorized the National Commission for the Protection of Human Subjects of Biomedical and Behavioral Research (the National Commission) in 1974 to study the use of helpless persons such as fetuses, children, prisoners, and the mentally ill in research, it also stipulated that the Department of Health, Education and Welfare (DHEW) would have to respond publicly to the National Commission's report.[3] In direct response to the report, DHEW promulgated regulations governing the use of human research subjects.[4]

Other commission reports, such as the report of the Ethics Advisory Board[5] created by the secretary of DHEW in 1978 to review funding applications for research involving human in vitro fertilization or other embryo research, were not as effective. The Ethics Advisory Board's report concluding that research on human embryos was ethically acceptable was tabled because of the political climate in 1979, and shortly thereafter DHEW disbanded the Board.[6] Regulations were promulgated in 1988[7] to reinstate the Board, but it was never formed.[8]

And yet other reports, such as those of the President's Commission for the Study of Ethical Problems in Medicine and Biomedical and Behavioral Research (the President's Commission), have had considerable influence even though Congress did not mandate any governmental agency to respond to the reports. The President's Commission was authorized by Congress in November 1978 to continue the earlier work of the National Commission and to consider numerous other issues in ethics and medicine.[9] Both government and private citizens took heed of the President's Commission's recommendations, particularly those regarding making decisions concerning withdrawal or withholding of medical treatment. The mere authority of its findings was accepted by other mechanisms for assuring accountability, and thus the President's Commission indirectly was very effective in shaping policy on several important issues.[10]

The Pros and Cons of Government Commissions as Mechanisms for Assuring Accountability

Expert Advice

The greatest advantage of government commissions is their potential for providing well-studied expert advice. Commissions can be comprised of some very knowledgeable members devoted to fully studying a problem and open to considering all possible solutions. Commissions often have full-time staffs and a multitude of government resources at their disposal, making a thorough investigation possible.

Some commissions have produced such comprehensive and well-thought-out reports that they have been widely accepted as authoritative both by government and private bodies, for example, the National Commission's and the President's Commission's reports. Even if one disagrees with some of the conclusions of these commissions, one must admit that their reports are very comprehensive.

Political Maneuvering

The very power that makes such an expert body possible can also cause good ideas to stagnate in a quagmire of political maneuvering. One example already discussed is the Ethics Advisory Board. In October 1977 the first in vitro fertilization funding proposal was approved by the National Institutes of Health,[11] but it was more than a year before the Board was formed and almost another year after that before a report was released, only to be ignored.[12] The battle over the Ethics Advisory Board reports continues.[13] Under these circumstances, the Ethics Advisory Board could be understood as a mere tool used by DHEW and later by DHHS to stall a politically difficult decision; when the Board came out with a recommendation that the administration did not like, it was simply ignored.

Another example of how politics can quagmire commissions is the congressionally authorized Biomedical Ethics Advisory Committee. After suffering from years of political struggle, the committee was, for all intents and purposes, disbanded when the congressional Biomedical Ethics Board in charge of appointing the committee was disbanded on 30 September 1990.[14] It could very well be that, although Congress could agree that such a committee was a good idea, once it came to actually determining the details of who should be on the committee and what its mandate should be, political disagreements prevented it from actually ever functioning.

In Summary

A commission of experts can help provide guidance for the assurance of accountability in various fields as long as such commissions actually are created and proceed with their work and are not used as an excuse for inaction. The National Commission and the President's Commission were extremely successful, but other examples such as the Ethics Advisory Board and the Biomedical Ethics Advisory Committee illustrate that sometimes commissions fail to do more than add to the frustration of those who would like to look to them for guidance. A very careful assessment of the political climate, or at least a willingness to simultaneously pursue other avenues, is required before placing one's confidence in the suggestions that a commission might make.

Commissions are weak mechanisms for assuring accountability. Their only enforcement power lies in the other mechanisms of accountability that adopt their suggestions and follow through on their implementation. Thus, although commissions may be a good beginning for studying accountability, they cannot be relied upon as a mechanism for enforcing accountability.

Where We Go From Here

There are even more types of mechanisms for assuring accountability than those described so far, but professional self-regulation, licensure and professional discipline, government contracts, judicial remedies, and government commissions are among the most applicable prototypes for assuring the accountability of bioethics committees and consultants. The one remaining flaw with my analysis is that it has concentrated on the accountability of individuals rather than groups of individuals. The next part seeks to rectify this failing by analyzing how two types of committees that could be seen as analogous to bioethics committees are held accountable.

PART THREE

The Accountability of Institutional Committees

Introduction to Part Three

The mechanisms described in part 2 dealt primarily with the accountability of individuals. Those mechanisms can serve as direct analogies for bioethics consultants, but it is not clear how such systems of accountability would apply to bioethics committees. To help illustrate how the part 2 mechanisms for assuring accountability apply to committees, this part examines the accountability of two other institutional committees that function within the medical context: institutional review boards (IRB) and peer review committees.

The reader should take care not to confuse the role IRBs and peer review committees play in holding medical professionals accountable with an analysis of how the committees themselves are held accountable. The latter is the focus of the discussion in this part.

Chapter Eight

Institutional Review Boards

There are several types of committees or boards involved in reviewing research. The National Institutes of Health (NIH) alone has at least half a dozen different types of committees, ranging from the less well-known data monitoring and safety boards to the far more familiar IRBs.[1] There is practically no information available on how the less well-known boards are monitored so, for the purposes of discussing accountability, we are warranted in limiting our analysis to the more familiar IRBs.

How Institutional Review Boards Work

The first federal requirement of committee review for research was a set of guidelines for research procedures established for the Clinical Center at NIH in 1953.[2] Committee review of proposed experimentation projects was an established practice in several medical schools as early as 1961.[3] In 1966, the Surgeon General of the United States Public Health Service (USPHS) published a policy statement requiring prior institutional review of research projects involving human subjects before the USPHS would approve funding for such research.[4] Since 1966 there have been several versions of the USPHS requirements, up until the present requirements under the Department of Health and Human Services (DHHS)[5] and the Food and Drug Administration (FDA).[6] These regulations parallel each other in most areas, but they differ in some respects.[7]

Under DHHS regulations, every institution involved in human research funded in any part by DHHS must have its research approved by an IRB.[8] Under FDA regulations, clinical investigations related to the substances FDA can regulate under the Federal Food, Drug, and Cosmetic Act must be approved by an IRB.[9] Both sets of regulations specify that the minimum number of members on IRBs is five, and that no board may be composed entirely of men or women, or of persons of one profession.[10] They also specify the procedures IRBs must follow in approving, modifying, or disapproving research proposals and for suspending or terminating of research projects.[11] The DHHS and the FDA have taken different approaches to assuring IRB accountability. The DHHS has established an accreditation process by which institutions negotiate with the NIH Office for Protection from Research Risks (OPRR) and offer the agency assurances that certain procedures will be followed.[12] Furthermore, there is the possibility of site visits from DHHS, and OPRR has undertaken the provision of educational programs to help assure the quality of IRB reviews.[13] FDA does not use the DHHS accreditation process; rather, it has implemented its own procedures for inspecting IRBs.[14] FDA inspections are not on-site peer review, but are surprise inspections by agents who know little, if anything, about what IRBs do.[15]

In addition to these types of agency review, the regulations allow for review by the institution for which the IRB functions.[16] Officials of the institution may disapprove research approved by an IRB, but they may not approve research that the IRB has disapproved.[17] While there is evidence that as many as forty-eight percent of the institutions with IRBs have established appeal procedures,[18] anecdotal evidence indicates that IRBs virtually never disapprove research projects and that requests for appellate review are rare.[19]

It is interesting to note that the mechanisms for assuring IRB accountability mentioned so far, as meager as they may be, are primarily due to yet another mechanism discussed in part 2. Public concern in the sixties and early seventies regarding the use of vulnerable human subjects in research led Congress to charge the National Commission for the Protection of Human Subjects of Biomedical and Behavioral Research (the National Commission) in 1974 to consider, among other things, the effectiveness of the IRB system of reviewing research proposals.[20] The National Commission sponsored studies to investigate IRB activities and the quality of their performance.[21] The results of these studies led to recommendations that the Department of Health, Education, and Welfare (DHEW), now DHHS, adopted almost without alteration and that served as the foundation for the regulations described in preceding paragraphs.

The last type of accountability available for IRBs is legal liability. IRBs do not have federally granted immunity. Some may be included under those state immunity statutes general enough to include a variety of hospital committees,[22] but in most states IRBs are without any special protection from liability. In principle, IRBs could be liable for all the different types of liability mentioned in part 2; however, IRBs have rarely been sued and, where they have been sued, complaints were dismissed or settled before any ruling on the merits was reached.[23] In the one reported case involving an IRB, *Head v. Colloton*,[24] the IRB's chairman was named as a defendant and the complaint sought an injunction to compel the IRB to amend a protocol involving bone marrow transplantation, but the case was resolved without addressing the issue of IRB liability.[25]

The Pros and Cons of How the Accountability of Institutional Review Boards Is Assured

National Standards and Federal Funding

The major advantage of treating bioethics committees like IRBs is that federal regulation could provide relatively clear and uniform requirements for all bioethics consultations. Some of the benefits of existing IRB regulations include guidelines for performing a risk/benefit analysis for the treatment proposed[26] and a means of ensuring that participants are suited for their role by, among other things, requiring informed consent.[27] Likewise, regulating the composition of bioethics committees the way IRB composition is regulated (that is, that the committee cannot consist of all women or all men or of persons from a single profession),[28] would help assure a degree of diversity that could prevent group biases from predominating. Also, as under existing IRB accountability controls, regular monitoring of bioethics committee and consultant activity by regulatory investigators could help ensure forthright deliberations.

If the analogy is drawn less stringently, the same types of regulations that govern IRBs would not be required for bioethics committees and consultants, but regulations could be specifically tailored to meet the objectives of bioethics consultation and could be promulgated independently of those regulations already in existence for IRBs. The pros and cons of such regulations would greatly depend on their content. For example, unlike IRB regulations, they could provide for explicit means of complaining about the procedures followed by committees or consultants, or they could provide for certain types of committee and consultant immunity from liability.[29] (Part 4 makes some more in-depth suggestions regarding the possible content of regulations.)

The most obvious disadvantage of the IRB analogy is that federal regulations require federal intervention. First, regulations must be linked to the federal spending power[30] or some other constitutionally granted authority[31] to pass constitutional muster.[32] Secondly, the federal government has been hesitant to become involved in clinical ethical dilemmas. In principle, these disadvantages could be overcome by having regulation imposed on the state level, as is being done in Maryland.[33] But, state action risks the loss of national uniformity and, as yet, the National Conference of Commissioners on Uniform State Laws has not shown any interest in creating a model law regarding bioethics consultation.

Accreditation and Site Checks

The methods of assuring accountability specified by the DHHS and the FDA may not be appropriate for bioethics committees and consultants. Accreditation is a form of review that only takes place at the funding stage of research; and a more continuous form of monitoring, such as investigations or site visits, could hamper the frankness of bioethics deliberations, particularly if there are no special safeguards to maintain confidentiality.

Self-Regulation and the Patient-Physician Relationship

Other less obvious disadvantages of the IRB analogy are that federal regulation creates a disincentive for the bioethics profession to exercise some form of self-control to assure the accountability of bioethics committees and consultants. The major advantage of encouraging the profession to monitor itself is that such a system creates a closer knit and less intrusive form of review, with each individual being aware of his or her responsibilities and encouraging responsible activity in others. It also promotes professional integrity and a sense of pride in professional standards, both of which could encourage more general compliance than government regulation.

Lastly, there are some commentators who argue that bioethics committees and consultants may be a mistake because they interfere with the patient-physician relationship in decision making, or because they might take the role of ethical decision making out of the hands of the patient, the patient's family, or another guardian or proxy.[34] This point should not encourage us to abandon bioethics consultation, but rather to regulate it, so that decision-making authority remains with patients, their families, friends, or surrogates, and their physicians.[35] However, the more removed the mechanisms of accountability are from understanding the medical setting, the more caution will have to be exercised to assure that regulations do not unnecessarily intrude on the patient-physician relationship.

In Summary

IRBs are held accountable through federal regulations requiring accreditation or on-site checks and the possibility of commission or court review. These mechanisms for assuring the accountability of IRBs are not frequently employed, but perhaps they are not employed because IRBs are functioning well without such oversight. On the other hand, due to constitutional and other constraints, it may be easier to implement regulatory guidelines for how bioethics consultations should be granted and conducted on the state level rather than the federal level.

Where We Go From Here

Our discussion of the regulation of IRBs has given us an insight into how government regulation of committee functions can help provide for accountability. The next chapter will give us some insight into how private regulation can help assure the accountability of institutional committees. Chapter 9 discusses peer review committees and how they are affected by private regulation and the potential for legal liability.

CHAPTER NINE

Peer Review Committees

Unlike IRBs, the mechanisms in place to assure the accountability of peer review committees are primarily private. The potential for court intervention, however, has had a strong influence on how peer review is conducted and just recently has stimulated the passage of federal laws protecting peer review committees from certain types of liability.

How Peer Review Committees Work

A Brief Definition

Peer review committees are formed within medical institutions to review and monitor the work of that institution's medical professionals. The committees consist primarily of professionals who have either volunteered or been appointed to the task by institutional administrators. Peer review committees are not the same as Professional Standards Review Organizations (PSRO) or Peer Review Organizations (PRO). The former are created by the hospitals themselves, usually under their bylaws, in accordance with the guidelines provided by the Joint Commission on Accreditation of Healthcare Organizations (Joint Commission).[1] The latter type of organization, created in accordance with federal law, reviews the quality of care of all hospitals that serve Medicare or Medicaid patients.[2] PSROs and PROs were discussed in chapter 5.

Professional Self-Regulation: The Joint Commission Mandate

The Joint Commission requires hospitals to perform peer review that is intended to help advance a medical institution's own quality control.[3] To carry out this peer review, institutions usually organize committees that may have a variety of names; for simplicity's sake they will be referred to here as peer review committees.[4] The Joint Commission regulates a variety of types of health-care facilities, but this section will concentrate on its regulation of hospitals.

The Joint Commission has set out standards requiring that "each clinical department or major clinical service (or medical staff, for a nondepartmentalized medical staff) holds monthly meetings to consider findings from the ongoing monitoring and evaluation of the quality and appropriateness of the care and treatment provided to patients."[5] An older version of these standards specifies that "[s]uch mechanisms shall be designed to maintain high professional standards of care."[6] These controls are usually enforced by departmentalized committees. For example, some committees will monitor the quality of surgical procedures;[7] others will ensure that patients' records are accurately kept;[8] and still others will investigate the credentials of applicants for staff positions and consider when those privileges should be revoked or suspended.[9] The composition of peer review committees is not specified by the Joint Commission; however, it can be assumed that they are primarily, if not exclusively, composed of health-care professionals. It should also be noted that membership on such committees is voluntary, uncompensated work,[10] and that evaluating a colleague's performance and possibly having to instigate disciplinary action is probably not a pleasant task.

Given these factors, we should not be surprised that peer review committee activities are easily hampered by a threat of litigation. The possibility of becoming embroiled in legal disputes can discourage physicians from volunteering to work on such committees. And, even if enough members are assembled, the threat of liability may discourage frank and open discussion. In principle, such committees are susceptible to at least seven types of legal liability: defamation, antitrust violations, interference with practice of profession, breach of contract, interference with contractual relations, negligence, and violation of due process.[11]

Government Intervention

Professional self-regulation is reinforced in all states by laws requiring and/ or protecting the peer review process.

Laws Requiring Peer Review

Many states mandate or encourage the use of peer review committees in medical institutions. For example, in Massachusetts every licensed hospital must have an established program for investigating, reviewing, and resolving reports of physician incompetence.[12] In Arizona, statutes specify that committees or other organizational structures for monitoring quality assurance are required in all state health-care institutions, but are optional in other institutions.[13] And in still other states professional societies are either mandated[14] or provided with the option[15] of establishing peer review committees.

Laws Protecting the Peer Review Process
At the State Level

A concern for intraprofessional quality control has led all states to adopt some form of limitation on the liability of peer review committees. Historically, the protections provided have ranged from absolute immunity from civil suit to qualified immunity only for defamation actions.[16] However, the immunity statutes are qualified to require peer review committee members to act reasonably,[17] without malice,[18] or in good faith.[19]

In certain institutions, there may also be immunity from liability for committee members if they are seen as being institutional officers in a jurisdiction where that institution is protected by either a sovereign or charitable immunity.[20] Concern regarding the openness of committee deliberations has led some states to limit the degree to which committee proceedings can be obtained during discovery.[21] The provisions, however, do not necessarily correspond with the immunity from civil suit provisions.[22]

At the Federal Level

The federal government has also recently taken steps to protect peer review procedures. The Health Care Quality Improvement Act of 1986, enacted 14 November 1986,[23] was Congress's answer to peer review participants' complaints about the possibility of being sued for treble damages in actions for antitrust violations.[24] The act's protections, however, are strictly limited both in their provision of immunity from civil liability[25] and in their provision for the confidentiality of peer review deliberations.[26]

The act's immunity provision applies to persons acting with respect to professional review actions for professional review bodies.[27] Of particular relevance is that the immunity provision applies only to private actions, does not affect state or federal enforcement power, and specifically does not protect against civil rights actions.[28] The immunity provision is also only effective if the act's requirement for reporting peer review actions against physicians to the Secretary of DHHS is followed.[29] Furthermore, the immunity provided, as in many states,[30] only creates a presumption that peer review actions are protected from liability.[31] A showing by the preponderance of the evidence that any of the following criteria have not been met will defeat the presumption of immunity:

Professional review action must be taken
(1) in the reasonable belief that the action was in the furtherance of quality health care
(2) after a reasonable effort to obtain the facts of the matter
(3) after adequate notice and hearing procedures are afforded to the physician involved or after such other procedures as are fair to the physician under the circumstances

(4) in the reasonable belief that the action was warranted by the facts known after such reasonable effort to obtain facts and after meeting the requirement of (3).[32]

The act's confidentiality provision protects peer review reports made to the Secretary of DHHS and state medical boards.[33] The act also establishes a national registry of disciplined physicians and requires that peer review committees report to state boards any action that adversely affects a physician's clinical privileges for a period of over thirty days.[34] State medical boards in turn must make reports to the Secretary of DHHS.[35] The secretary will make reports available to organizations considering physicians for employment or in the case of disciplinary actions or malpractice suits.[36] Similarly, information in the hands of peer review committees or state disciplinary boards is confidential except with reference to reporting requirements specified in the act, professional review activities, and malpractice litigation.[37]

The Pros and Cons of How the Accountability of Peer Review Committees Is Assured

Delicate Topics

Peer review committees serve as a good analogy for bioethics committees and consultants because many of the problems with which peer review committees deal are as sensitive as those dealt with by bioethics committees and consultants. Peer review committees evaluate the qualifications and ongoing work of health-care professionals.[38] Whether or not someone is qualified to get or maintain a job is certainly a delicate topic. Publication of the opinions of committee members could damage either their reputations or the reputations of the professionals they evaluate. Publication of the deliberations of bioethics committees or consultants could have the same damaging effects, particularly if a committee or consultant makes disparaging remarks regarding someone's character or life history. Thus, some of the types of protections warranted for peer review committees may also be warranted for bioethics committees and consultants.

For example, it may be appropriate to grant bioethics committees and consultants the same types of immunities, both from liability and from discovery, that are granted peer review committees by some states or by the federal Health Care Quality Improvement Act.[39] Such protections would help assure the confidentiality of patient records or committee members' and consultants' opinions and could prevent ethical issues from being debated in the sometimes hostile, adversarial setting of court litigation.

A Need for Some Court Review

The obvious disadvantage of this peer review analogy is that, in some states, the assurance of accountability through the courts has been all but eliminated. This is particularly problematic if bioethics committees and consultants are granted practically absolute immunity as is the case in Maryland.[40] Society should not want to leave the resolution of ethical dilemmas to committees and consultants whose deliberations are secret and who are only kept in check by their hospitals or professional organizations. An appeal to hospital officials or some other interested organization such as a professional organization seems a meager form of recourse for someone who feels his or her rights have been violated. Limiting accountability review to such organizations cuts an aggrieved party off from any traditional avenues of seeking remedies for a wrong committed. Moreover, under the peer review analogy, complaining parties would probably have no more right to access consultation deliberations than anyone else, so they would not have a means of substantiating whether or not their rights actually had been violated. Such protections may give bioethics committees and consultants an unjustifiable amount of power and a license to act without concern for procedural fairness; they could make decisions based on unacceptable biases, and there would be no mechanism, or only a very limited one, for reviewing the grounds for their recommendations.

In Summary

Peer review committees are held accountable by private accreditation as well as by court-enforced liability. Unlike the other mechanisms discussed so far, the mechanisms used to assure the accountability of peer review committees illustrate how state and federal laws can check the overburdensome effects of the court intervention.

Where We Go From Here

With this chapter on peer review committees, we have completed our analysis of possible mechanisms to use as prototypes for assuring the accountability of bioethics committees and consultants. The next step is to discuss, in more detail, the possible application of these mechanism for assuring accountability to bioethics committees and consultants. That is the undertaking of part 4.

PART FOUR

Assuring the Accountability of Bioethics Committees and Consultants

Introduction to Part Four

With the first two tasks of this book behind us, it is now time to apply the principles we have learned in part 1 and the examples we have explored in parts 2 and 3 to develop an accountability scheme appropriate for bioethics committees and consultants. Part 4 is not a model law or policy for holding bioethics committees and consultants accountable; rather, it is a description of the fundamental considerations that any such law or policy would need to address. This book concludes that it is time to implement some form of mechanism for holding bioethics committees and consultants accountable. Preferably, such a mechanism will be developed by or with significant input from those presently involved in bioethics consultation. Whatever the frame work developed to implement the accountability of bioethics committees and consultants, the issues raised in this part should be carefully considered in shaping the specifics of such a mechanism.

CHAPTER TEN

The Accountability Scheme

One unfortunate aspect of our political system is that sometimes the more controversial a topic, the less likely it is to be regulated. Bioethical issues involve questions that in many respects are very private, but in other respects are of the utmost concern for society as a whole. Dying is a very personal experience, yet how and when patients decide to die or when health-care personnel decide a life is no longer worth saving is of great social concern. The few times that government has become directly involved in regulating such topics have resulted in severe criticism. (Consider the Baby Doe regulations,[1] and the Supreme Court's decisions in *Cruzan v. Director, Missouri Department of Health*,[2] and *Webster v. Reproductive Health Services.*[3])

Bioethics committees and consultants have become a type of pressure valve, providing a means to resolve bioethical disputes without the need to resort to government agencies or the courts. This is a development welcomed by most. The more these issues can be resolved amicably, the better. But society should be interested in what bioethics committees and consultants do and how they give advice. When society sanctions such activities, it should want them to be conducted fairly. The imposition of mechanisms of accountability, whether by private or public institutions, could help to assure procedural fairness.

The General Goal of Procedural Fairness

This book does not pretend to provide answers for the myriads of difficult bioethical questions facing our society today; rather it suggests that a uniform application of general principles of procedural due process through mechanisms for assuring accountability would make bioethics consultation more equitable. I am not suggesting that the content of bioethics consultation be regulated to the extent that the activities of professionals are regulated, but only that procedures be implemented to help assure some fairness in how bioethics consultations are granted and conducted. Such procedures could help prevent the arbitrary loss of individual freedoms, such as the freedom to act in accordance with one's religious beliefs, the freedom not to suffer unwarranted discrimination, and the freedom to make one's own health-care decisions. Unfortunately, there is the grave possibility that, without procedural safeguards, bioethics committees and consultants will violate such freedoms more frequently than we would like.

These goals are aspirational; I do not argue that there is any legal mandate for implementing mechanisms to assure due process as there is for government. My primary motivation for suggesting the implementation of accountability mechanisms is to improve the bioethics consultation process. Professional self-interest, however, should also motivate those involved in bioethics consultation to advocate the imposition of mechanisms for assuring the accountability of bioethics committees and consultants. Bioethics consultation is a new field that lacks credibility and guidance. If each consultation is pursued differently, potential clients may receive the impression that bioethics committees and consultants do not know what they are doing. Uniformity of process can help prevent this impression. Accountability also helps create confidence in a profession by indicating that there is supervision of bioethics consultation services and a concern for fair treatment. And finally, mechanisms of accountability can provide guidance for those interested in pursuing a career in bioethics consultation and thereby improve the quality of services provided.

The Particular Goal of Holding Bioethics Committees and Consultants Accountable

This section discusses how the mechanisms of accountability discussed in parts 2 and 3 could be applied to bioethics consultation services.

Professional Self-Regulation

Effective professional self-regulation is probably the best way to assure accountability. Professional self-regulation allows those with the greatest knowledge of the process of bioethics consultation to establish guidelines, set standards, evaluate performance, and take disciplinary action. If self-regulation is effective, government intervention and cost to the taxpayer can be kept at a minimum. Court involvement would still be necessary when there are breaches of existing laws, but a need for regulatory guidance could be eliminated, thus keeping the private sector in control of professional regulation.

Those involved in bioethics consultation should seriously consider creating some professional mechanisms for assuring their own accountability. Such regulation would bring credibility to the profession and provide clients with confidence in bioethics consultation by assuring them that there is some supervision of the services they are provided. Professional self-regulation might also preempt potentially disastrous government intervention. Those involved in bioethics consultation might not have enough control over the political process to assure that measures imposed are based on accurate assessments, present realistic expectations, and provide adequate guidance. Government might not feel a need to regulate bioethics committees and consultants if those involved in bioethics consultation have set their own standards; or government regulation, if it does take place, may rely heavily on the standards developed within the profession.

The primary problem with professional self-regulation by those involved in bioethics consultation is that the field is new enough that there is considerable disagreement among practitioners as to the goals and process of bioethics consultation, or even as to the value of self-regulation. Members of the Society for Bioethics Consultation have hotly debated the issue of professional self-regulation for years. Most concerns, however, center on the difficulty of setting substantive rather than procedural standards. Perhaps an emphasis on setting only procedural standards could make professional self-regulation more palatable to those already in the profession. If not, efforts to implement self-regulation may have to begin among a smaller group of professionals.

Standard-Setting Organizations

Some of those already involved in bioethics consultation could create a professional organization interested in setting guidelines and/or disciplining its members. Both types of organizations could help fashion procedural reports or guidelines, certifying bioethics consultants or accrediting bioethics consultation services and educational programs for those interested in becoming involved in bioethics consultation. A group with open membership would have the advantage of not excluding anyone from the debate, while a membership organization with disciplinary jurisdiction is likely to be more effective at assuring the implementation of its suggestions. There is no reason why both types of organizations could not have an overlap in membership and work together to the advantage of both organizations and the profession.

Even if government acts to regulate bioethics consultation, private organizations could hold their members to more exalted standards. As a Joint Commission on Accreditation of Healthcare Organizations president has stated, organizations like the Joint Commission should be the "standard-bearer[s] of *high*-quality health care."[4] Similarly, organizations formed by those involved in bioethics consultation could do much to improve the standing of their profession.

Publication

Publication would also be a possible way of assuring the accountability of bioethics committees and consultants, but it is a mechanism that probably needs to be implemented in conjunction with others to be effective. A voluntary system of publication might be useful for the exchange of information, but it probably would not provide much accountability. It is even likely, due to the expense and time involved in preparing minutes or case reports for publication, that little material would be submitted for publication. One can imagine a bioethics journal including some interesting case reports for the consideration and comment of its readers, but it is difficult to imagine that a journal devoted to nothing but the publication of such reports would have enough of a readership to support the cost of publication.

Publication as a requirement imposed through another mechanism for assuring accountability is more likely to be a successful means of monitoring bioethics committee and consultant activities, yet even then it would be reasonable to limit the type of publication expected. For example, a membership organization, or government regulatory body, could require that minutes or case records be available for public scrutiny, or alternatively, publication could be limited to organizational members or even review staff trained to look for procedural deficits. Under these conditions, the activities of bioethics committees and consultants could be subject to public or peer criticism without all the disadvantages of journal publication.

Even a more limited type of publication might be difficult to accomplish because of the cost involved in maintaining records and editing them to preserve patient confidentiality. While it may be commonplace for bioethics committees to have someone taking minutes at their meetings, efforts would still need to be made to edit those minutes to protect patient confidentiality. It is even less likely that an individual consultant, or small team of consultants, will have the time to write up and edit reports for every consultation. Requiring such reports may take precious time away from more important efforts, such as educating health-care personnel on bioethical issues and doing consultations.

As a possible compromise, the types of consultations that needed to be reported in detail could be limited. For example, only formal meetings would need to be reported, and access to case reports and committee minutes could be limited to specific persons in charge of conducting peer review, who would be allowed to look at unedited reports.

Licensure and Professional Discipline

As bioethics consultation becomes a more established profession, government licensure and discipline may become inevitable. At this point, however, such licensure, in the traditional sense of requiring proof of minimum competency discussed in chapter 4, could be detrimental to the profession. Even those involved in bioethics consultation services are unclear regarding what type of qualifications committees and consultants should have. Unless requirements are drawn so widely that licensure does not require any special skills, some people with potentially valuable contributions to make to the field would be excluded. Licensure might be appropriate if carried out in a nontraditional way by requiring, as a condition for licensure, only that specified procedural safeguards are respected. As long as requirements are well considered and enforcement is actually carried out, such licensure could be a welcome development on the state level. Unfortunately, in Maryland, the one state where bioethics committees are explicitly regulated,[5] enforcement authority rests with a state medical board that barely has enough time to deal with disciplining medical professionals, let alone bioethics committees.[6] Thus, if states take action to assure the accountability of bioethics consulting services, one would hope there is enough commitment to the project that adequate resources are allocated for enforcement.

And finally, as with all government regulation, those involved in bioethics consultation should be leery of well-meaning politicians and bureaucrats who are not well informed on the issues relevant to bioethics committees and consultants. Thus, efforts at professional self-regulation would be both in the interest of the general public and those involved in bioethics consultation services, because professional organizations could set standards and provide government with guidance should government regulation become inevitable.

Government Contracting

Government contracting is a viable possibility for assuring the accountability of bioethics committees and consultants. If done at the federal level, such regulation would have to be tied to the government's spending power. The requisite spending authority could be established, as it is for Peer Review Organizations, by making compliance with review procedures a condition for institutional participation in the Medicaid and Medicare programs.

The only disadvantages of this approach are those that apply to all forms of government regulation. Such programs must be carried out at public expense and may not be sensitive to professional realities. Government contracts may be difficult to develop if there has not been some organized effort to determine exactly what procedures should be required of bioethics consultation services. A government contracting scheme that is developed with the benefit of sufficient input from those involved in bioethics consultation could satisfy both professional and societal needs. It would be best if such regulation could be developed with the benefit of a professional organization's or government commission's report on specific requirements for holding bioethics committees and consultants accountable.

Judicial Remedies

A very practical aspect of the accountability problem is that it is unclear when, if at all, bioethics committee members and consultants could be held liable for their advice. To date, there is only one instance of a bioethics committee being sued; and there are no instances of a bioethics consultant being sued. Elizabeth Bouvia, a quadriplegic suffering from cerebral palsy, who refused the insertion of a nasogastric feeding tube, sued the bioethics committee at the hospital that disregarded her refusal and advising her physicians that she should be force fed.[7] Interestingly, her attorney, Richard Scott, a physician himself, has stated: "I'm not against ethics committees. I think they're helpful, and I think more hospitals should have them. But I don't think that an ethics committee should have any right to make or inflict decisions on people *and not be held accountable for it any more than anybody else*."[8] Although Bouvia's suit for damages was dismissed without ever deciding the issue of bioethics committee liability,[9] it is clear that bioethics committees and consultants are vulnerable to lawsuits.

At first it may seem that it would be more appropriate to use the potential liability of peer review committees as a model for the liability of bioethics committees, and the potential liability of physician consultants as a model for bioethics consultants. Yet, the types of functions performed by peer review committees make them susceptible to types of litigation not relevant to the activities of a bioethics committee. In addition to suits for negligence, peer review committees are susceptible to suits for violation of due process, antitrust, interference with practice of profession, breach of contract, and interference with contractual relations.[10] Violations of due process, strictly speaking, do not apply to bioethics committees and consultants because, unlike peer review committees, which are mandated by law, bioethics committees and consultants do not perform government-type functions necessitating compliance with constitutional principles of due process. All the other types of suits are related to a peer review committee's function of evaluating the work of physicians and deciding whether or not their staff privileges should be denied or revoked or if their behavior should be reported to state or federal authorities for disciplinary action. Bioethics committees and consultants give advice--they do not make decisions in the sense that peer review committees do. Furthermore, the interests at stake in peer review committee decisions are economic in nature, thus creating all the possible tort actions for interference with economic rights. Bioethics committees and consultants do not generally deal with questions of economic rights.

Malpractice

A better analogy for both bioethics committees and consultants is the independent physician consultant who is called in to assist the treating physician with the analysis of a special problem. The advice given by this physician can be negligently given if it does not meet the standard for average, competent advice for the physician's specific expertise. Similarly, if a committee holds itself, or a consultant holds him or herself, out to be an expert in a specific area (bioethical issues), the advice given should meet some average level of competence.

For a committee, this standard might mean that at least some members of the committee research the topic at issue or that the committee only deal with issues on which it has educated itself in the past. It might mean that a committee should not give advice until it has taken the time to set up certain procedural standards for doing consultations or until all its members have received a very basic education on bioethical issues and the process of ethical decision making. For a consultant, the same rules would apply, but, in addition to clinical experience, a consultant's competence could also be assessed by his or her degree of formal training in ethics.

Liability for negligence greatly depends on whether the case was handled fairly and in an acceptable manner. Formalized procedures for handling bioethics consultations that are, in fact, followed can help protect both bioethics committees and consultants against liability. For a committee, such protections may be implemented by fulfilling quorum requirements, allowing every committee member present a chance to comment, and providing as much time as possible for a thorough consideration of the issues at hand. For bioethics committees and consultants, adequate procedures might include a standard method for collecting relevant information, contacting relevant parties, examining the patient's chart, following a specific process for distinguishing legal, medical, and ethical issues, and accurately documenting the consultation.

Particularly relevant to our inquiry is that a theory of bioethical malpractice would depend on a measurable standard of skill and care that could be expected from the average prudent member of the profession.[11] For physicians, this standard is based on what can be expected of the average competent physician;[12] what constitutes competency can be derived from minimum standards established by the profession itself.[13] In the absence of clear standards, the court will determine what is expected. To help preempt such a court determination, bioethics committees and consultants may wish to set standards themselves.

Fiduciary Principles

Another type of liability that may develop is one based on fiduciary principles, such as those governing a director's obligations to his or her corporation, but caution must be taken not to draw the analogy too closely. It is important to note that the majority rule is that corporations are only obligated to consider the interests of the corporation,[14] even though some corporate statutes extend directors' obligations to include the interests of customers and the community where the corporation is located.[15] If a direct analogy is made to bioethics committees and consultants, this would mean that bioethics committees and consultants would owe their fiduciary duties to the medical institutions for which they work. But the accountability at issue here is accountability to groups further removed from the actual delivery of health care, such as professional organizations or government bodies.

Moreover, as discussed in chapter 6, when acting outside the realm of their fiduciary duties to the corporation, directors are not held to any exacting standard of care--they are subject to the regular negligence standard[16] of the ordinary prudent person discussed in the next section. So for the fiduciary duty analogy to work in the bioethics consultation context, the law would have to clearly define what authority medical institutions can or cannot give bioethics committees or consultants. In other words, the law would still have to decide whether it is within an institution's discretion to allow its bioethics committee or consultant to give advice on the basis of unacceptable factors such as race or social status. If the law allows such considerations and the hospital authorizes or ratifies advice based on such considerations, then, under the corporate director-ship analogy, the bioethics committee's or consultant's actions would be pro-tected as within their discretion. But, if certain considerations are prohibited by law or the institution, then the bioethics committee or consultant would be acting *ultra vires* in giving advice based on those considerations and would be subject to liability as would any nonprofessional.

A very important implication of fiduciary principles is that the regulation of bioethics committee and consultant deliberations need not originate in the law. Fiduciary principles can be contractually based; for example, corporations, clients, or grantors have an explicit or implied agreement with corporate directors, attorneys, or trustees that their activities will be conducted in a certain manner.[17] Medical institutions and, perhaps, professional organizations for bioethics committees and consultants could require bioethics committees and consultations to be handled in a specified manner. Those specifications could then be incorporated into the law as part of a bioethics committee's and consultant's fiduciary duties to the medical institutions, the profession, or society.

Some Other Theories of Liability

In addition to malpractice or fiduciary liability, bioethics committees and consultants could be liable for several other types of wrongs. Bioethics commit-tees and consultants could be liable for ordinary negligence. To avoid liability for ordinary negligence, a person must act in the manner that a reasonable, prudent person in his or her situation could be expected to act; no expertise is assumed.[18] For example, absent any higher standard, one can imagine a bioethics commit-tee or consultant being held liable for negligence because he or she did not exercise the reasonable care a prudent person would have exercised in collecting or reviewing documents before giving their advice.

Bioethics committees and consultants could also be liable for the torts of intentional infliction of emotional distress and defamation. Intentional infliction of emotional distress requires that an actor's extreme and outrageous, inten-tional, or reckless conduct causes severe emotional distress in another.[19] One could imagine a bioethics committee's or consultant's advice that someone is unfit to participate in an organ transplant program (for example, because of his or her emotional makeup or personal history) could cause severe emotional distress. The only problem would be proving that such distress was intentional or recklessly caused.[20] To prove that a bioethics committee or consultant defamed someone by advising against his or her inclusion in an organ transplantation program, one would have to show that there was a communication to third parties and that the communication was one tending to injure "reputation" in the commonly understood sense of that word: that what was communicated tended to injure esteem, respect, good will, confidence, or excite derogatory or unpleasant feelings or opinions against the plaintiff.[21]

Outside the realm of torts, bioethics committees and consultants could be liable for civil rights violations or even conspiracy to commit criminal acts. Civil rights[22] are protected by federal and state constitutions, and by legislation passed by Congress or the states.[23] Depending somewhat upon the jurisdiction in which a remedy is sought, actions could be brought against a bioethics committee or consultant for advice given under the pretext of ethical reasoning, that was actually based on unjustifiable considerations of race, age, religion, sex, marital status, or other unacceptable forms of discrimination.[24] One very real impetus for such litigation might be the Civil Rights Commission's recent report stating that the practice of denying life-sustaining treatment to disabled infants is a violation of federal antidiscrimination laws.[25]

Finally, bioethics committees and consultants could, although it is not very likely, be guilty of conspiracy to commit a crime.[26] Conviction for conspiracy requires a showing of partnership in criminal purpose with the actual perpetrator of the crime. A bioethics committee, its members, or a consultant would have to knowingly agree with the criminal intent of the person carrying out the criminal act to be guilty of conspiracy.[27] The difficulty in proving such conspiracy would lie in the requirement of *criminal* intent. There must be an agreement to commit an unlawful act.[28] If a bioethics committee member or bioethics consultant inadvertently gave advice that leads to a criminal act, that person could be guilty of negligence, but not conspiracy. Thus, the fear I have sometimes heard expressed, that those involved in bioethics consultation could be found guilty of murder without having intended any harm, is completely unfounded.

Some General Comments

Courts provide individualized review and remedies tailored to the specific damages that were suffered. Courts are open in their investigations and attempt to bring to light all relevant facts, allowing for a thorough debate on the merits of a particular complaint. Unlike in the case of intra-professional review, the decision makers have no personal stake in the outcome of the decision. Similarly, courts should be isolated from political motivations that may influence a government regulatory review process.

Some of the very advantages of court enforcement are also its disadvantages. The accountability of bioethics committees and consultants is such a new and unusual problem that it may be wrong to try to deal with it under a system of legal principles intended and adapted to serve in totally different contexts. Existing principles may not be suited for dealing with the unique problems caused by bioethics consultation. For example, by what criteria would a court determine the duties and standards involved in a suit for ethical malpractice? Would not the possibility of such suits discourage people from volunteering to serve as members of bioethics committees or as bioethics consultants? Or, how could a court proceeding function effectively without bringing all the very private problems faced by patients into public view? And would not such publicity discourage open and frank discussions during bioethics consultations? As we have seen in chapter 9, these types of concerns induced many legislatures to grant peer review committee members various degrees of immunity from liability and from discovery. Perhaps such protections could also be granted bioethics committees and consultants.

Limiting Liability
Bioethics committees and consultants could be protected from some forms of liability through the passage of a statute such as the federal Health Quality Improvement Act. Obviously, antitrust liability is not as great a concern for bioethics committees and consultants as it is for peer review committees; although bioethics committees and consultants may influence peer review proceedings, it is not their responsibility to evaluate professional performance. On the other hand, a need for confidentiality and openness during consultations is a concern bioethics committees and consultants share with peer review committees. Although a statute like the federal Health Quality Improvement Act is justified by the federal interstate commerce power to regulate antitrust actions, it is not clear what justification would serve for passing such an act with respect to bioethics committees and consultants. Thus, it is probably preferable to pass legislation on the state level. State laws could set procedural standards for bioethics consultations and prevent most unwarranted suits by raising the burden of proof the plaintiff must meet in order to sue successfully. Perhaps a uniform law on the subject should be considered by the National Conference of Commissioners on Uniform State Laws. It is, however, important to note that such laws should not absolutely preclude all types of liability and that they should not alter the burden of proof for civil rights violations or criminal actions. These latter exceptions are essential, because not even the smooth running of bioethics consultations is sufficient grounds to justify hampering someone's ability to be heard in court when the charges are as grave as civil rights or criminal violations.

Even if a regulatory scheme is devised to assure accountability, the possibility of individualized adjudication should not be precluded. Regulations, including site-checks, are primarily preventive measures. Court actions can also provide compensation to those who are injured. This type of restitutionary measure is hard to achieve without some type of adjudication, albeit administrative adjudication is an option.

Government Commissions

Probably the best beginning in an effort to develop structures for assuring the accountability of bioethics committees and consultants would be a consideration of the issues involved by a government commission. Although we may agree that some form of accountability for bioethics committees and consultants is desirable, the details of how such accountability should be assured still need much consideration. Having people knowledgeable in both the practical and theoretical aspects of bioethics consultation and in other fields such as law, health care, and political science come together, with sufficient resources to make a concerted effort to resolve issues of how the accountability of bioethics committees and consultants should be assured, would be ideal.

Such a commission could avoid some of the disadvantages of other mechanisms we have discussed. One hopes that political and professional concerns would not predominate over the more general needs of society and that a well-thought-out report with realistic suggestions would result. One disadvantage of this mechanism is that logically, it is only a first step. For its recommendations to have effect, they would need to be enforced either through private or government regulation.

Some Possible Specific Requirements for Holding Bioethics Committees and Consultants Accountable

In an earlier draft of this book, I tried to sketch out some of the details of what types of procedures should be required for granting and carrying out bioethics consultations. My success in that regard was limited because currently there is no empirical evidence to justify choosing one set of procedures over another. Although I have some first-hand experience with several bioethics consultation services, this is not a book in the social sciences, and an empirical study of how bioethics committees and consultants function is beyond its scope. With this limitation in mind, this section includes some general comments regarding the types of requirements that might be appropriate for assuring the accountability of bioethics committees and consultants.

There are six types of issues that need to be addressed when considering specific requirements for assuring the procedural fairness of bioethics consultation, whether done by committees or consultants: (1) access, (2) training, (3) proceedings, (4) documentation, (5) peer review, and (6) appeal procedures.

Additionally, there is a seventh issue that should be addressed only with regard to bioethics committees, namely the composition of such committees.

Access

One very important aspect of procedural fairness involves issues of equal access. There should be some uniformity regarding who has access to bioethics consultations and under what circumstances consultations are granted. Unfortunately, the access issue is treated very differently by different consultation programs. There are two aspects to the access question. One is the question of who may call a consultation, and the other is a question of who may attend consultations. Some programs provide consultations only upon a physician's request and usually allow only physicians to attend; others allow more liberal access, calling consultations at the request of a wide variety of interested persons and inviting anyone involved in the patient's care to attend.

Bioethics consultation is a service potentially valuable to a wide range of persons, and thus no one involved in a patient's care should be excluded. Allowing all relevant interested persons to initiate or attend a bioethics consultation will increase the chances that problems will be resolved without anyone's feeling that he or she was unjustifiably excluded.

Irrespective of who is allowed access, the rules should be applied consistently in as large a group of medical institutions as possible. Whether regulation is imposed through private organizations or government, access issues should be treated the same in all regulated institutions; the goal being to achieve enough uniformity that people know what to expect and to obviate arbitrary denials of service.

Other aspects of access should also be considered. There should be some form of screening process to assure that consultations actually involve ethical issues, and referrals for medical and legal advice should be made to those qualified to give such advice. Questions regarding who should be invited to attend consultations must also be decided. Just as it would be unfair to allow patients to request consultations in some cases and not in others, it would be unfair in some cases to invite everyone involved and not to do the same in all similar situations. To allow arbitrary treatment creates the possibility that unacceptable factors are being considered in determining who should be invited. For example, a relevant person's personality, religious beliefs, age, race, or sex may play a role in whether members of a bioethics consultation team want him or her present. Uniform notice and request-for-attendance requirements would make such discrimination more difficult.

Having access requirements does not mean that, in every case, everyone needs to be notified and included in deliberations. Some distinctions could be made between different types of consultations. For example, notification requirements could be different for "formal" versus "informal" consultations, or for emergency or bedside consultations and others. Also, emergency consultations may prevent notification of more than a few of the most relevant persons because of time constraints. Regardless of how such distinctions are drawn, equal access should be assured for each category of consultation.

Training

Both bioethics committees and consultants should meet minimum training requirements. For committees, this could mean that all committee members or core committee members must have some very basic training in identifying and resolving ethical issues. This could mean that they must attend a formal program like the University of Virginia Center for Biomedical Ethics Fellows Program, or the Georgetown University Kennedy Institute of Ethics Intensive Bioethics Course. Or, it could mean that they only need to read and familiarize themselves with standard materials suggested or provided by a regulating body. Alternatively, individual committee members would not be required to satisfy any training requirements, but at least one committee member would have to meet certain requirements such as qualifying as a certified bioethics consultant. Of course, both a qualified consultant and some educational requirements for all committee members would also be an option.

For consultants, the requirements could be as minimal as reading basic materials in bioethics or as comprehensive as requiring formal university training in ethics. Other possible requirements could include a basic knowledge of clinical terminology and different philosophical or religious tenets. In addition to, or instead of, formal educational requirements, some form of on-the-job training with a qualified bioethics consultant or clinical program could be required.

Proceedings

One would not want to dictate exactly what types of proceedings are followed during a bioethics consultation because much would depend on the circumstances, but some specific requirements should be imposed. For example, some sort of fact finding should be required. A committee member or the bioethics consultant should be required to familiarize him or herself with the facts by speaking with the attending physician, the patient, family members, and social workers and/or by reading the patient's chart. Ideally this investigation should take place between the request for a consultation and when the consultation is given, but again, circumstances such as an emergency may make more than a brief discussion with the attending physician or a glance at the patient's chart an unrealistic expectation.

It may also be advisable to require that each consultation begin with a statement that clearly delineates the limits of bioethics consultation. An effort should be made to remind participants that bioethics committee members and consultants do not adjudicate disputes and that they are not qualified (unless they are also licensed attorneys) to give legal advice. The role of bioethics consultation is to give ethical advice. Who the ultimate decision maker is, be it the patient or someone else, is dictated by law.

Another procedural requirement might be some means of assuring that everyone has an opportunity to speak. Often nonphysician health-care personnel or patients and their families are intimidated by physicians or by the very fact that a consultation is taking place. Procedural safeguards assuring a chance to speak could help participants overcome some of their fears of contributing to bioethics consultation proceedings.

Documentation

Documentation is advisable because it creates a record for future reference. It may even be advisable, from a legal standpoint, to require a notation in a patient's chart that a consultation took place and a brief summary of the advice given. Such documentation may prevent confusion as to what was done and serve as notice to anyone who is involved with the patient's care who did not attend the consultation.

Documentation is essential if any form of publication is required. Accurate records are also crucial for any type of retroactive evaluation of how bioethics consultations are conducted. Of course, whenever documentation is prepared for the consideration of persons other than those directly involved in patient care, precautions should be taken to protect patient confidentiality.

Peer Review

Some form of peer review should exist, whether it is carried out through publication or through spot-checks by designated reviewers. Due to confidentiality problems, it would probably be preferable that whatever mechanism is implemented to assure accountability provide some form of organized peer review. Specially designated personnel could review records, sit in on consultations, and report deviations from accepted procedural practices to the regulating agency.

Appeal Procedures

The possibility that someone directly involved in bioethics consultation may wish to draw attention to possible procedural misconduct should not be dismissed. The regulating organization should provide a procedure by which complaints are heard and acted upon. Perhaps complaints could trigger a spot-check or other form of investigation into the procedures followed by a bioethics consultation service. Efforts could even be made to correct wrongs immediately, for example, by requiring a consultation with someone improperly denied access to consultation services.

Composition

Finally, for bioethics committees, a regulatory body may consider making certain requirements regarding committee composition. Both medical boards and peer review committees have traditionally been dominated by male physicians. There is also some evidence that bioethics committees are currently dominated by physicians. Such skewed representation on committees may not be optimal for assuring that this society's plurality of ethical perspectives is respected. As has been achieved with the regulation of institutional review board composition, some efforts should be made to diversify the composition of bioethics committees and thereby minimize the likelihood that certain types of biases will pervade bioethics deliberations.

Bioethics committees should include both health care personnel and persons not directly affiliated with the medical institution. The committee should not consist totally of persons trained in medicine. The type of health care personnel serving on the committee should depend on the type of institution and the interest of specific members of the health care community in being on the committee. If the institution specializes in a particular type of treatment, a physician who specializes in that treatment should be on the committee. In addition to a physician there should be a nurse, a social worker, a patient representative or chaplain, an attorney, and, if possible, a bioethicist.

The proper community member for inclusion on the committee may also depend on the type of institution. A parent with an ill or handicapped child might be helpful for a children's hospital. Otherwise, a former patient may be helpful or a concerned community member who understands or is willing to learn about bioethics consultation.

The attorney on the committee should not be the attorney who represents the institution because of possible conflicts of interest. In-house counsel is obligated to protect the institution's legal interests, and such interests could be in direct conflict with his or her role on the committee. For example, hospital counsel has no obligation to inform a patient of his or her right to take legal action against the hospital or its staff. Some would even say hospital counsel has an obligation not to disclose such information to the patient. However, an attorney who does not represent the institution, but who is knowledgeable on the law relevant to bioethical issues, could be a valuable asset on the committee. The attorney would be there not to give legal advice, but simply as a resource for what the law is, if there is any, on the particular topic at issue.

The committee should consist of a core group of five to ten dedicated people to keep meetings manageable. Others could be invited to educational sessions that interest them or to consultations regarding patients with whom they have dealt. Finally, specifications as to quorum requirements are advisable to prevent the opinion of one or two members from being misunderstood as representative of committee views.

In Summary

The accountability of bioethics committees and consultants can probably be best assured through a combination of the mechanisms discussed in parts 2 and 3. The best beginning would be a study of bioethics committee and consultant accountability issues by a government commission. Then the commission's findings, if satisfactory, could be adopted by private organizations or government in deciding what specific procedural standards bioethics committees and consultants should be required to satisfy. Some possible requirements to help assure procedural fairness have been discussed, particularly measures to assure equal access to bioethics consultations, adequate training, fair proceedings, documentation, peer review, appeal procedures, and the diversity of bioethics committee members. The implementation of such measures by an effective mechanism for assuring accountability would help improve bioethics consultation services by providing procedural safeguards that make bioethics consultation a more equitable process.

CONCLUSION

Bioethics consultation is a valuable service. There is no doubt that as time goes on and the profession of bioethics consultation grows, regulation is inevitable. Most professionals shun regulation, but certain types of regulations should be encouraged by those involved in bioethics consultation. The assurance of the accountability of bioethics committees and consultants could be carried out not by interfering with the substantive development of bioethics issues and how they are resolved, but by interjecting a modicum of order and fairness into how bioethics consultations are granted and conducted. Such regulation would add credibility to the profession and give potential clients more confidence in how bioethics consultations are handled. If carried out by the profession itself, such regulation could also forestall more intrusive and constraining government regulation.

This book has suggested three levels of control for assuring the accountability of bioethics committees and consultants. First, government commissions and/or professional organizations should study the appropriateness of certain procedural safeguards for improving the fairness of bioethics consultation services. The guidance provided should at least consider questions of access to bioethics consultation services, the training of bioethics committee members and consultants, how consultations should proceed and be documented, peer review, appeals procedures, and the composition of bioethics committees. Second, guidelines should be implemented through mechanisms responsive to professional needs, but not driven by economic interests. A professional organization could serve that purpose as long as the interest of its members and society coincide; otherwise government regulation would be preferable. Third, the possibility of court review should not be foreclosed. The threat of potential litigation could be stemmed, to some extent, by providing a rebuttable presumption of tort immunity for bioethics committees and consultants. This policy would discourage lawsuits but still permit review where the plaintiff can show the bioethics committee or consultant acted in bad faith, with criminal intent, or in violation of civil rights laws.

My personal experience with bioethics consultation services has ranged from great admiration for the professional handling of cases to shock over how some people with no training or experience can be functioning as institutional bioethics consultants, or how some committees function as little more than a forum for social interaction. I have seen the concerns of some individuals be ignored because they are old, young, women, or health-care personnel other than physicians. And I have seen consultations take place without the knowledge of key decision makers such as the patient, the attending physician, or a patient's surrogate. I hope this book will spark some interest in the further study of how bioethics committees and consultants should be held accountable and help us work toward well-run, effective, and fair bioethics consultation services.

REFERENCES

Chapter 1

1   See *Webster's New World Dictionary of the American Language*, 2nd ed., s.v. *account* and *accountability*.

2   See Aristotle, *Nichomachean Ethics*, trans. Terence Irwin (Indianapolis: Hackett Publishing Co., 1985); G.E.M. Anscombe, *Intention* (Ithaca, NY: Cornell University Press, 1969); D. Bennett, "Action, Reason, and Purpose," *Journal of Philosophy* 62 (4) (18 February 1965): 85.

3   See Aristotle, *Nichomachean Ethics*; J. Hospers, *Human Conduct* (New York: Harcourt, Brace & World, 1961).

4   See A. Souter, ed. *Texts and Studies*, Vol. IX, *Pelagius' Expositions of the 13 Epistles of St. Paul* (Cambridge: Cambridge University Press, 1926); T. Aquinas, "*Summa Theologica*" in *Introduction to Saint Thomas Aquinas*, ed. A.C. Pegis (New York: Random House, Inc., 1945); W.T. Stace, *Religion and the Modern Mind* (New York: Harper and Row, 1952).

5   See J. Glover, *Responsibility* (New Jersey: Humanities Press, 1970); J. Rawls, "Two Concepts of Rules," Part I, *Philosophical Review* LXIV (1955): 3-13.

6   The dichotomy established here is an imperfect one. *Social* accountability, although distinct from *moral* accountability, should not be misunderstood as not involving questions of morality. All theories of accountability, even those described here as social, fall within the realm of ethical or moral theory.

7   See Aristotle, *Nichomachean Ethics*.

8   See Anscombe, *Intention*.

9   See R. Taylor, *Metaphysics*, 2nd ed. (Englewood Cliffs, NJ: Prentice-Hall, Inc., 1974).

10 See C.D. Broad, *The Mind and Its Place in Nature* (London: Routledge & Kegan Paul, Ltd., 1925).

11 See R. Taylor, "Causation," *Monist* 47 (1963): 287.

12 See generally Aristotle, *Nichomachean Ethics*; I. Kant, *Foundations of the Metaphysics of Morals*, trans. L.W. Beck (Indianapolis: Bobbs-Merrill Co., Inc., 1959); Aquinas, *Summa Theologica*; A.C. Ewing, *The Definition of Good* (New York: Macmillan Co., 1947).

13 See T. Szasz, *Law, Liberty and Psychiatry* (New York: Macmillan Co., 1963).

14 See H.L.A. Hart and A.M. Honoré, *Causation in the Law* (Oxford: Oxford University Press, 1959).

15   See H.F. Pitkin, *The Concept of Representation* (Berkeley: University of California Press, 1967).

16   See H.L.A. Hart, *The Concept of Law* (Oxford: Oxford University Press, 1961).

17   See R. Dworkin, *Law's Empire* (Cambridge, MA: Belknap Press, 1986).

18   See C.B. MacPherson, *Democratic Theory: Essays in Retrieval* (Oxford: Clarendon Press, 1973).

19   See M. Walzer, *Spheres of Justice* (New York: Basic Books, 1983).

20   See Pitkin, *The Concept of Representation*; J.H. Ely, *Democracy and Distrust: a Theory of Judicial Review* (Cambridge, MA: Harvard University Press, 1980).

21   See R. Nozick, *Philosophical Explanations* (Cambridge, MA: Belknap Press of Harvard University Press, 1981).

22   See F.D. Schoeman, "On Incapacitating the Dangerous," *Philosophical Quarterly* 16 (1) (1979).

23   See Nozick, *Philosophical Explanations*; R.E. Barnett, "Restitution: A New Paradigm of Criminal Justice," *Ethics* 87 (4) (July 1977): 279; D.A. Conway, "Capital Punishment and Deterrence: Some Consideration in Dialogue Form," *Philosophy and Public Affairs* 3 (4) (Summer, 1974): 431; H. Morris, "Person and Punishment," *Monist* 52 (4) (October 1968): 475.

24   The "before-the-fact/after-the-fact accountability" distinction is borrowed from G.J. Agich, "The Concept of Responsibility in Medicine," in *Responsibility in Health Care*, ed. G. Agich (Boston: Dordrecht, Holland, Co., 1982), 60, note 7.

25   Although regulating procedures can affect the substantive outcome of bioethics consultations, such effects would be minimal compared to the direct regulation of the content of advice and are an unavoidable consequence of improving the bioethics consultation process.

26   See J.C. Fletcher, "Standards for Evaluation of Ethics Consultation," in *Ethics Consultation in Health Care*, eds. J.C. Fletcher, N. Quist, A.R. Jonsen (Ann Arbor, MI: Health Administration Press, 1989), 173-184.

27   See generally, Aristotle, *Nichomachean Ethics*.; T. Irwin (Indianapolis: Hackett Publishing Co., 1985); Kant, *Foundations of the Metaphysics of Morals*; Aquinas, *Summa Theologica*; Ewing, *The Definition of Good*.

28   See generally, J.S. Mill, "On Liberty," in *John Stuart Mill: A Selection of His Works*, ed. J.M. Robson (Indianapolis: Bobbs-Merrill Co., Inc., 1966); G.R. Semin and A.S.R. Manstead, *The Accountability of Conduct: A Social Psychological Analysis* (New York: Academic Press, 1983).

29   H.T. Engelhardt, Jr., *The Foundations of Bioethics* (New York: Oxford University Press, 1986), 12.

30   *Ibid.*

31   *Ibid.*, 32.

Chapter 2

1   *In re Quinlan*, 355 A.2d 647 (NJ), *cert. denied. sub nom. Garger v. New Jersey*, 429 US 922 (1976).

2   President's Commission for the Study of Ethical Problems in Medicine and Biomedical and Behavioral Research, *Deciding to Forego Life-Sustaining Treatment: Ethical, Medical and Legal Issues in Treatment Decisions* (Washington, DC: U.S. Government Printing Office, 1983), 155-65 [hereinafter *Deciding to Forego Treatment*].

3   Department of Health and Human Services, "Nondiscrimination on the Basis of Handicap; Procedures and Guidelines Relating to Health Care for Handicapped Infants; Final Rule," *Federal Register* 49 (16 January 1984): 1621-1654.

4   MD Health-Gen. Code. §§ 19-370 to 19-374 (1990).

5   Senator John C. Danforth introduced a bill on 17 October 1989 providing for a Patient Self-Determination Act of 1989 mandating, among other things, the establishment of Institutional Ethics Committees (S.1766). This aspect of the Act was not included in the House version introduced by Representative Sander Levin on 3 April 1990 (H.R. 5067) and the provision mandating bioethics committees was not included in the bill that passed on 26 October 1990 as part of the Budget Reconciliation Act of 1990. 42 U.S.C. 1395cc(a)(1): Medicare Provider Agreements Assuring the Implementation of a Patient's Right to Participation in and Direct Health Care Decisions Affecting the Patient.

6   Joint Commission on Accreditation of Healthcare Organizations, *1992 Hospital Accreditation Manual* (Chicago: Joint Commission, 1992), RI1, RI2.

7   S. J. Youngner, D. L. Jackson, C. Coulton, *et al.*, "A National Survey of Hospital Ethics Committees," in *Deciding to Forego Treatment*, 443, 446.

8   D. J. Guido, "Hospital Ethics Committees: Potential Mediators of Educational and Policy Change," *Dissertation Abstracts International* 43 (Michigan: University Microfilms International, 1983), 3529.

9   A.L. Otten, "Ethics Experts Help More Doctors Handle Hard Moral Decisions," *The Wall Street Journal* (6 March 1987): 1, col. 1; D.D. Dine, "Ethics Panels Multiplying to Grapple with Tough Issues," *Modern Healthcare* (14 October 1988): 22.

10   Otten, "Ethics Experts Help More Doctors Handle Hard Moral Decisions," 1, col. 1. For a discussion of the discrepancies in survey reports regarding the number of ethics committees, see R. E. Cranford and A. E. Doudera, "The Emergence of Institutional Ethics Committees," *Law, Medicine & Health Care* (February 1984): 11.

11   See Judicial Council Report, "Guidelines for Ethics Committees in Health Care Institutions" *Journal of American Medical Association* 253 (1985): 2698 (ethics committee members should be primarily health care professionals); D.

Avard, G. Griener, and J. Langstaff, "Hospital Ethics Committees: Survey Reveals Characteristics," *Dimensions in Health Service* 62 (February 1985): 24, 25 (Canadian survey reveals diverse committee composition with general emphasis on health-care providers); C. Levine, "Hospital Ethics Committees: A Guarded Prognosis," *Hastings Center Report* 7 (June 1977): 25, 27 (report from conference at Hastings Center suggests participants felt physicians were over-represented on ethics committees).

12 K. Murphy, "Malpractice Allegation Is Added to Bouvia's Lawsuit," *Los Angeles Times* (8 October 1986): p. 3, col. 1.

13 It is quite common for hospitals to have one major consultant who then organizes and calls committee meetings when necessary. Charles Culvert is one such person. Otten, "Ethics Experts Help More Doctors Handle Hard Moral Decisions"; Dine, "Ethics Panels Multiplying to Grapple with Tough Issues"; John Fletcher served a similar function while at the National Institutes of Health. Interview with J. Fletcher, 6 February 1987.

14 *Ibid.*

15 See generally J.M. Gibson and T.K. Kushner, "Will the 'Conscience of an Institution' Become Society's Servant?" *Hastings Center Report* 16 (June 1986): 8; *Deciding to Forego Treatment*, 160-165; Department of Health and Human Services, "Service and Treatment for Disabled Infants; Model Guidelines for Health Care Providers to Establish Infant Care Review Committees," *Federal Register* 50 (15 April 1985): 14893; Cranford and Doudera, "The Emergence of Institutional Ethics Committees," 16-17; R.E. Cranford, F.A. Hester, and B.Z. Ashley, "Institutional Ethics Committees: Issues of Confidentiality and Immunity," *Law, Medicine, & Health Care* 13 (April 1985): 52, 52-53; C.G. Ferguson, "Medical Ethics Committees--The Decision is Yours," *Dimensions in Health Service* 61 (September 1984): 36, 39.

16 M.R. Wicclair, "The Distinction Between Medical and Ethical Decisions," in *Ethics in the Hospital Setting*, ed. Bruce Weinstein (Morgantown, WV: West Virginia University Press, 1985), 16-17 (discussing patients' tendency to rely on medical professionals for advice in all aspects of health care, even ethical advice).

17 R.M. Veatch, *A Theory of Medical Ethics* (New York: Basic Books, Inc., 1981), part 1 (discussing various medical traditions and codes of practice).

18 For example, R.M. Veatch, "Courts, Committees, and Caring," *American Medical News*, 23 (23 May 1980); Impact/1-Impact/2+ (discussing how bioethics committees might interfere with the patient-physician relationship); A. Browne, "Ethics Committees for What?" (editorial) *Canadian Medical Association Journal* 36 (11) (1 June 1987): 1149-1151 (suggesting that the role of bioethics committees be severely limited).

19 *Ibid.*

20 R.A. McCormick, "Ethics Committees: Promise or Peril?" *Law, Medicine and Health Care* 12 (September 1984): 150-155.

21 *Ibid.*

22 J.F. Fletcher, *Situation Ethics: The New Morality* (Philadelphia: Westminster Press, 1966).

23 For example, McCormick, "Ethics Committees: Promise or Peril?" 153-54 (criticizing bioethics committees for their lack of expertise).

24 F. Rosner, "Hospital Medical Ethics Committees: A Review of Their Development," *Journal of the American Medical Association* 253 (10 May 1985): 2693, 2695 (advocating the use of bioethics committees as a means of avoiding liability); R.E. Cranford and A.E. Doudera, *Institutional Ethics Committees and Health Care Decision Making* (Ann Arbor, MI: Health Administration Press, 1984), 52-54 (same).

25 M. Siegler, "Ethics Committees: Decisions by Bureaucracy," *Hastings Center Report* 16 (June 1986): 22.

26 Veatch, "Courts Committees, and Caring"; McCormick, "Ethics Committees: Promise or Peril?"

27 *Ibid.*

28 Plato, *The Republic* in *The Dialogues of Plato*, Vol III, trans. with analyses and introductions by B. Jowett (New York: Oxford University Press, 1892); Aristotle, *The Politics of Aristotle*, trans. E. Barker (London: Oxford University Press, 1977); Hobbes, *Leviathan*, ed. C.B. Macpherson (Middlesex: Penguin Books, 1968); J. Locke, *Two Treatises of Government*, introduction and notes by P. Laslett (Cambridge: Cambridge University Press, 1960).

29 See Pitkin, *The Concept of Representation*; C.J. Friedrich, "The Dilemma of Administrative Responsibility," in *Responsibility*, ed. C.J. Friedrich (New York: Liberal Arts Press, Inc., 1960), 152-170, 189-202; F.H. Knight, "Political Responsibility in a Democracy" in *Responsibility*, ed. C.J. Friedrich, 171-88.

30 S.H. Kadish, "Methodology and Criteria in Due Process Adjudication--A Survey and Criticism," *Yale Law Journal* 66 (1956-57): 319, 340.

31 J. Rawls, *A Theory of Justice* (Cambridge, MA: Harvard University Press, 1971), 85.

32 *Ibid.*

33 *Ibid.*

34 *Ibid.*, 197-98, 221-24. See also J. Rawls, "Kantian Constructivism in Moral Theory," *Journal of Philosophy* 77 (September 1980): 515-577.

35 Dworkin, *Law's Empire*.

36 *Ibid.*, 164.

37 *Ibid.*, 165.

38 *Ibid.*, 165-66.

39 *Ibid.*, 167.

40 *Ibid.*, 167-77.

41 *Ibid.*, 178.

42 *Ibid.*, 179.

43 *Ibid.*, 178-184, 206-208.

44 *Ibid.*
45 *Ibid.*, 185.
46 *Ibid.*
47 *Ibid.*
48 *Ibid.*, 179.
49 *Ibid.*, 179, 219.
50 *Ibid.*, 183-84.
51 *Ibid.*, 184.
52 *Ibid.*, 185.
53 *Ibid.*, 223.
54 *Ibid.*, 215.
55 *Ibid.*, 185-86.
56 See *ibid.*, 178.
57 See *ibid.*
58 See *ibid.*, 166, 174-75.
59 See *ibid.*, 164.
60 See *ibid.*, 178-186.
61 The Maryland Bar Association is considering the possibility of suggesting to the Maryland legislature that bioethics committee decisions be binding in cases involving incompetent patients who have left no advance directives and have no family members to look after their interests. Conversation with D. Hoffmann, Assistant Professor of Law and Healthcare at the University of Maryland School of Law, on 2 August 1990.

Chapter 3

1 L.S. King, "The Founding of the American Medical Association," *Journal of the American Medical Association* 248 (8 October 1982): 1749.
2 *Ibid.*
3 N.S. Davis, *History of the American Medical Association from Its Organization up to January 1855*, ed. S.W. Butler (Philadelphia: Lippincott, Grambo & Co., 1855), 135, 139.
4 *Ibid.*
5 W.T. Reich, ed., *Encyclopedia of Bioethics*, Vol. 3 (New York: Free Press, 1978), under the word "Medical Profession, Part II-Organized Medicine," by J.G. Burrow.
6 *Ibid.*
7 R.C. Derbyshire, *Medical Licensure and Discipline in the United States* (Baltimore: Johns Hopkins Press, 1969), 89.
8 F.D. Campion, *The AMA and U.S. Health Policy Since 1940* (Chicago: Chicago Review Press, 1984), 46-47.
9 *Ibid.*
10 Other organizations include: the Association of American Medical Col-

leges, the American Board of Medical Specialties, and the Coordinating Council on Medical Education. See Karen Backus, ed., *Encyclopedia of Medical Organizations and Agencies*, 3rd. ed. (Detroit: Gale Research Inc., 1990).

11 Campion, *The AMA and U.S. Health Policy Since 1940*, 427.

12 National Science Foundation, *Self-Regulation in the Professions: Accounting, Law, Medicine*. Principal investigator H.L. Shuchman (Glastonbury, CT: Futures Group, July 1981).

13 *Ibid.*

14 F.P. Grad and N. Marti, *Physicians' Licensure and Discipline: The Legal and Professional Regulation of Medical Practice* (Dobbs Ferry, NY: Oceana Publications, Inc., 1979), 8.

15 M. Friedman, *Capitalism and Freedom* (Chicago: University of Chicago Press, 1962), 149-60.

16 *Ibid.*, 150.

17 *Ibid.*

18 *Ibid.*, 152-53.

19 *Ibid.*

20 *Ibid.*, 154.

21 National Science Foundation, *Self-Regulation in the Professions: Accounting, Law, Medicine*, 180-81.

22 American Hospital Association, "AMA Stymies Patient 'Bill of Rights'," *Hospital Ethics* 6 (1) (January/February 1990): 4. A Bill of Rights was later approved at the AMA's June 1990 meeting. V. Cohn, "AMA to Members: Put Patients First," *Washington Post Health Section*, 13 November 1990, 12.

23 *Health Policy Week* 19 (24) (25 June 1990): 1.

24 *Ibid.*

25 *Ibid.*

26 Derbyshire, *Medical Licensure and Discipline in the United States*, 13-17.

27 See *ibid.*

28 See *ibid.*

29 Campion, *The AMA and U.S. Health Policy Since 1940*, 50.

30 Derbyshire, *Medical Licensure and Discipline in the United States*, 13-17.

31 American Board of Medical Specialties, *Directory of Medical Specialties: 1979-1980*, 19th ed., vol. 1 (Evanston, IL: Marquis Who's Who, 1979), xviii.

32 National Science Foundation, *Self-Regulation in the Professions: Accounting, Law , Medicine*, 199.

33 *Ibid.*

34 *Ibid.*

35 *Ibid.*

36 *Ibid.*

37 *Ibid.*, 201.

38 Grad and Marti, *Physicians' Licensure and Discipline: The Legal and Professional Regulation of Medical Practice*, 91.

39   For example, the American Boards of Dermatology, Orthopaedic Surgery, Otolaryngology, Psychiatry, and Neurology.

40   For example, the American Boards of Dermatology, Radiology, and Thoracic Surgery.

41   For example, the American Boards of Anesthesiology, Obstetrics, and Gynecology.

42   For example, the American Boards of Family Practice and Urology.

43   "Board Certification and Physicians' Income," *Pro Forum* 1 (1) (June 1978): 4. See also for a more recent mention of this same phenomenon "Focus on Medical Specialists: Credentialing the Superspecialist," *Staff Privileges Report* III (3) (July 1990): 5-6.

44   National Science Foundation, *Self-Regulation in the Professions: Accounting, Law Medicine*, 210.

45   *Ibid*.

46   *Ibid*.

47   *Ibid*.

48   L.S. King, "The Founding of the American Medical Association," 1749.

49   Campion, *The AMA and U.S. Health Policy Since 1940*, 46-47.

50   *Ibid*.

51   *Ibid*.

52   *Ibid*., 49.

53   Mill, "On Liberty," 21-71.

54   *Ibid*.

55   *Ibid*.

56   F.K. Murphy and H.B. Dull, "Identification of Patients," (letter) *Annals of Internal Medicine* 79 (6) (December 1973): 907.

57   C. Morgan, "Confidentiality in Case-Reports," (letter) *Lancet* 1 (8429) (16 March 1985): 644.

Chapter 4

1   Department of Health, Education, and Welfare, *Report on Licensure and Related Personnel Credentialing* (Washington, DC: U.S. Government Printing Office, 1971), 7.

2   Grad and Marti, *Physicians' Licensure and Discipline*, 1.

3   TN Code Ann. §§ 63-2, 63-101 to 63-127; §§ 4-507 to 4-527 (1986).

4   *Ibid*.

5   NY Pub. Health Law § 230 (McKinney 1985 and 1990 Supp.); NY Educ. Law §§ 6509, 6511 (McKinney 1985 and 1990 Supp.).

6   For example, Wisconsin, WI Stat. Ann. § 15.405 (7) (West 1986).

7   Grad and Marti, *Physicians' Licensure and Discipline*, 20-22.

8   MD Health Occupations Code Ann. § 14-202 (1986). 1988 amendments

shifted this responsibility to the governor. MD Health Occupations Code Ann. § 14-202 (1989 Supp.).

9   AL Code § 22-2-1 (1984).

10 Grad and Marti, *Physicians' Licensure and Discipline*, 58.

11 The categories listed here are an adaptation and update of the list provided by Grad and Marti in *Physicians' Licensure and Discipline*, 120-21.

12 National Science Foundation, *Self-Regulation in the Professions: Accounting, Law, Medicine*. Principal investigator H.L. Shuchman (Glastonbury, CT: Futures Group, July 1981), 229.

13 *Ibid.*

14 E. Friedson, *The Profession of Medicine: A Study of the Sociology of Applied Knowledge* (Chicago: University of Chicago Press, 1970).

15 R.J. Feinstein, "Special Report: The Ethics of Professional Regulation," *The New England Journal of Medicine* 13 (2) (21 March 1985): 801.

16 Derbyshire, *Medical Licensure and Discipline in the United States,* 89.

17 Breaden and Balusha's article, "Official 1985 Federaton Summary of Reported Disciplinary Actions," in the *Federation Bulletin* (October 1986): 300, provided the figures for the number of physicians disciplined to calculate the averages given and the AMA's book, *Physician Characteristics and Distribution in the U.S.* (Chicago: American Medical Association, 1986), 8, gave the total number of licensed physicians used to calculate the averages given.

18 The Health Care Quality Improvement Act of 1986, 42 US Code 11101 to 11152, created the National Practitioner Data Bank, which went into effect on 1 September 1990. This data bank was created to help those involved in the provision of medical services or disciplining medical professionals identify incompetent performance or unprofessional conduct by medical professionals. It is too early to tell whether reporting requirements will be circumvented or whether the data bank will effectively provide interested parties with the data they need to make informed decisions about hiring or disciplining medical professionals.

Chapter 5

1   Social Security Act, § 1861(k)(1), 42 U.S.C. § 1395x(k)(1) (1982 and 1989 Supp.).

2   The Social Security Amendments of 1972, Pub. L. No. 92-603, § 249F.

3   § 1155(a)(1) as created by the Social Security Amendments of 1972, repealed by the Tax Equity and Fiscal Responsibility Act of 1982, Title XI-B of the Social Security Act, Pub. L. No. 97-248 (TEFRA) §§ 1151 *et seq.*, 42 U.S.C. §§ 1320c *et seq.* (1982 and 1989 Supp.).

4   A.G. Gosfield, ed. *1989 Health Law Handbook* (New York: Clark Boardman Co., Ltd., 1989), 363.

5   Tax Equity and Fiscal Responsibility Act of 1982, Title XI-B of the Social Security Act, Pub. L. No. 97-248 (TEFRA) §§ 1151 *et seq.*, 42 U.S.C. §§ 1320c *et seq.* (1982 and 1989 Supp.).

6   *Ibid.*

7   Social Security Act, § 1866(a)(1)(F), 42 U.S.C. § 1395 cc(a)(1)(F) (1982 and 1989 Supp.).

8   Gosfield, *1989 Health Law Handbook*, 364.

9   *Ibid.*

10   Department of Health and Human Services, "Medicare and Medicaid Programs; Utilization and Quality Control Peer Review Organizations (PRO); Assumption of Medicare Review Functions and Coordination with Medicaid, Final Rule," *Federal Register* 50 (17 April 1985): 15312-15374.

11   Department of Health and Human Services, "Medicare and Medicaid Programs; Changes to Peer Review Organizations Regulations, Proposed Rule," *Federal Register* 53 (16 March 1988): 8654-8667. As of February 1992 this proposal had not been finalized.

12   Gosfield, *1989 Health Law Handbook*, 365.

Chapter 6

1   The term "tort" is difficult to define because it includes a large number of unique types of civil, rather than criminal, wrongs that are not contractual for which a court can provide remedies. Torts can range from those that are intentionally inflicted to those that are due to negligent conduct. Battery, assault, infliction of emotional distress, trespass, negligence, nuisance, misrepresentation, and defamation are a few common torts.

2   W.P. Keeton, D.B. Dobbs, R.E. Keeton, and D.G. Owen, *Prosser and Keeton on the Law of Torts*, 5th ed. (St. Paul, MN: West Publishing Co., 1984), 164-165.

3   *Ibid.*

4   *Ibid.*

5   *Ibid.*

6   *Ibid.*

7   *Oliver v. Brock*, 342 So.2d 1, 3(AL 1976).

8   *Ibid.*

9   *Sullenger v. Setco Northwest*, 702 P.2d 1139, 1140-41 (OR App. 1985).

10   *Niccoli v. Thompson*, 713 S.W.2d 579, 583-84 (MO App. 1986).

11   *Ibid.*

12   *McCutcheon v. The Arch Diocese of Washington* (Mont. County Cir. Ct. 1988). This information was obtained from Bruce Adelson, one of plaintiff's counsel.

13   253 CA Rptr. 97 (1988).

14   675 P.2d 226, 231 (WA 1984) *(en banc)*.

15 But note that *in dicta* the court reserved the possibility that a malpractice action may be appropriate if a clergyman's failure to conform to church standards of care resulted in injury. *Ibid.*, 231.

16 K.B. Davis, "Judicial Review of Fiduciary Decisionmaking: Some Theoretical Perspectives," *Northwestern University Law Review* 80 (1985): 1 (discussing theory of fiduciary duties and giving examples in various professions).

17 H.G. Henn and J.R. Alexander, *Laws of Corporations and Other Business Enterprises*, 3d. ed. (St. Paul, MN: West Publishing Co., 1983 and 1986 Supp.) § 235; Revised *Model Business Corp. Act* §§ 8.01, 8.11, 8.30 (1984).

18 *Ibid.*

19 *Litwin (Rosemarin) v. Allen*, 25 N.Y.S.2d 667, 677 (Sup. Ct. 1940). This type of language is quite common in fiduciary cases. Davis, "Judicial Review of Fiduciary Decisionmaking: Some Theoretical Perspectives," 102 (discussing language used to describe fiduciary duties).

20 For example, *Graham v. Allis-Chalmers Manufacturing Co.*, 188 A.2d 125 (Del. 1963) (directors must recklessly respond with confidence to an obviously untrustworthy employee's information for there to be liability for passive negligence).

21 For example, *Francis v. United Jersey Bank*, 432 A.2d 814 (NJ 1981) (defendant, who by virtue of her office could have prevented the depredation of other insiders, had a duty to prevent such loss).

22 Henn and Alexander, *Laws of Corporations and Other Business Enterprises*, § 242.

23 *Ibid.*

24 Keeton, *Prosser and Keeton on the Law of Torts*, 54-65.

25 *Ibid.*, 773-74.

26 See generally H.J. Abraham, *Freedom and the Court: Civil Rights and Liberties in the United States*, 4th ed. (New York: Oxford University Press, 1982) (discussing various types of civil rights protections); L.H. Tribe, *American Constitutional Law* (Mineola, NY: Foundation Press, 1978), 256-275 (same).

27 *Ibid.*

Chapter 7

1 See L. Walters, "Commissions and Bioethics," *Journal of Medicine and Philosophy* (Special Issue: Bioethics Commissions: International Perspectives) 14 (4) (August 1989): 363-4. This article also includes a discussion of the historic development of commissions. For a discussion of how commissions have functioned in the United Kingdom, Australia, Canada, France, Germany, and Japan see *ibid.* pp. 369-472.

2 L. Walters, "Commissions and Bioethics," 364-65 (educating the government, as well as the public, is my own addition, although this possibility is not precluded by Walters's discussion).

3   Pub. L. No. 93-348, 88 Stat. 342 (12 July 1974).

4   Department of Health and Human Services, "Final Regulations Amending Basic HHS Policy for the Protection of Human Research Subjects," *Federal Register* 46 (26 January 1981): 8366-8401.

5   Department of Health and Human Services, "Ethics Advisory Board; Notice of Establishment," *Federal Register* 53 (12 September 1988): 35232.

6   *Ibid.*

7   *Ibid.*, 35232-33.

8   A 2 November 1989 letter from HHS Secretary Louis Sullivan to the National Institutes of Health states that the U.S. should not give the impression that it is supporting abortion by funding research on aborted fetuses, thus continuing the ban on such funding indefinitely. And, on 2 April 1989 Assistant Secretary of Health James Mason told the House Energy and Commerce Health Subcommittee that there definitely will be no federal funding for fetal tissue research. S. Fry-Revere, "Legal Trends in Bioethics," *The Journal of Clinical Ethics* (Summer 1990): 162. However, on 18 September 1990, Representative Henry Waxman introduced a bill (H.R. 5661) that, among other things, would end the current moratorium on federally funded fetal tissue research, and take the responsibility for regulating such research out of the hands of the secretary of HHS, and give it to ethics advisory boards. *Ibid.* (Spring 1991): 73. Efforts to lift the federal funding ban continued. By spring 1992, when this book went to press, the House had passed a bill lifting the ban, and the efforts to do the same in the Senate were gaining momentum. If Congress passes a bill, there still is the question of whether there is enough support to override President Bush's threatened veto.

9   Pub. L. No. 95-622, Title III, 42 U.S.C., Ch. 6A. A (1978).

10   For example, see the remarks of Representative Sander M. Levin upon the introduction of his version of the Patient Self-Determination Act that was passed on 26 October 1990. It cited the President's Commission report's discussion of advance directives as grounds for passing his bill. Congress, House, Representative Sander Levin introduced the Patient Self-Determination Act of 1990, *Congressional Record* (3 April 1990): E943.

11   L.R. Kass, *Toward a More Natural Science* (New York: Free Press, 1985), 100.

12   A.L. Bonnicksen, *In Vitro Fertilization: Building Policy from Laboratories to Legislatures* (New York: Columbia University Press, 1989), 77-79.

13   See note 8 of this chapter.

14   Conversation with Dr. Edmund D. Pellegrino, Vice Chairman of the Biomedical Ethics Advisory Committee, on 27 February 1990. See also A.M. Capron, "Bioethics on the Congressional Agenda," *Hastings Center Report* 19 (2) (March/April 1989): 22-23; and R.M. Cook-Deegan, "Abortion Politics Deals Death Blow to Bioethics Body Set Up by Congress," *Kennedy Institute of Ethics Newsletter* 4, no. 3 (3 July 1990): 3.

Chapter 8

1   DHHS has also promulgated guidelines for research involving recombinant DNA molecules that, in some cases, require the approval or research proposals by an Institutional Biosafety Committee. Department of Health and Human Services, "Guidelines for Research Involving Recombinant DNA Molecules; Notice," *Federal Register* 51 (7 May 1986): 16958-16985. The functioning of these committees is somewhat different than that of the DHHS and FDA IRBs, so, for simplicity's sake, my discussion will be limited to IRBs. For a description of Institutional Biosafety Committee membership and functions see *Ibid.* § IV-B, 16962-63.

2   National Institutes of Health, "Group Consideration for Clinical Research Procedures Deviating from Accepted Medical Practice of Involving Unusual Hazard," (17 November 1953), in R. Levine, *Ethics and Regulation of Clinical Research* (Baltimore: Urban and Schwarzenberg, 1981), 208. For pre-1953 developments see R. R. Faden and T. L. Beauchamp, *A History and Theory of Informed Consent* (New York: Oxford University Press, 1986), 200-201.

3   L. G. Welt, "Reflections on the Problems of Human Experimentation," in J. Katz, *Experimentation with Human Beings: The Authority of the Investigator, Subject, Professions and State in the Human Experimentation Process* (New York: Russell Sage Foundation, 1972), 889.

4   Levine, *Ethics and Regulation of Clinical Research*, 209.

5   Department of Health and Human Services, *Code of Federal Regulations* 45 (Washington, DC: U.S. Government Printing Office, 1989), § 46.

6   Food and Drug Administration, *Code of Federal Regulations* 21 (Washington, DC: U.S. Government Printing Office, 1989), § 50 (informed consent for human subjects), § 56 (operation of IRBs) (note: these are the major sections dealing with IRBs and experimentation on human subjects, but FDA rules on informed consent are spread out over a variety of sections on other topics); Levine, *Ethics and Regulation of Clinical Research*, 209-210.

7   For an account of how DHHS and FDA regulations vary, see D. M. Maloney, *Protection of Human Research Subjects: A Practical Guide to Federal Laws and Regulations* (New York: Plenum Press, 1984), 58-64. Also see Faden and Beauchamp, *A History and Theory of Informed Consent*, 202-215.

8   Department of Health and Human Services, *Code of Federal Regulations* 45 (Washington, DC: U.S. Government Printing Office, 1989), § 46.

9   Food and Drug Administration, *Code of Federal Regulations* 21 (Washington, DC: U.S. Government Printing Office, 1989), §§ 50, 56.

10   Department of Health and Human Services, *Code of Federal Regulations* 45 (Washington, DC: U.S. Government Printing Office, 1989), § 46.107; Food and Drug Administration, *Code of Federal Regulations* 21 (Washington, DC: U.S.

Government Printing Office, 1989), § 56.107. Also see Office of Science and Technology Policy, "Proposed Model Federal Policy for Protection of Human Subjects; Response to the First Biennial Report of the President's Commission for the Study of Ethical Problems in Medicine and Biomedical and Behavioral Research," *Federal Register* 51 (3 June 1986): 20204-20217 (these rules require "every nondiscriminating effort . . . to ensure that no IRB consists entirely of men or entirely of women. . . .").

11 Department of Health and Human Services, *Code of Federal Regulations* 45 (Washington, DC: U.S. Government Printing Office, 1989), §§ 46.109-113; Food and Drug Administration, *Code of Federal Regulations* 21 (Washington, DC: U.S. Government Printing Office, 1989), §§ 56.109-56.113.

12 Levine, *Ethics and Regulation of Clinical Research*, 239.

13 *Ibid.*

14 Food and Drug Administration, *Code of Federal Regulations* 21 (Washington, DC: U.S. Government Printing Office, 1989), §§ 56.120-56.121.

15 Levine, *Ethics and Regulation of Clinical Research*, 239.

16 Department of Health and Human Services, *Code of Federal Regulations* 45 (Washington, DC: U.S. Government Printing Office, 1989), § 56.112.

17 *Ibid.*

18 Cooke, "Tannenbaum & Gray, A Survey of Institutional Review Boards and Research Involving Human Subjects," in National Commission for the Protection of Human Subjects of Biomedical and Behavioral Research, *Report and Recommendations: Institutional Review Boards* (Washington, DC: U.S. Government Printing Office, 1978: DHEW Publication No. (OS) 78-0008), Appendix (1978). But see P. J. Greene, Durch, Horwitz and Hopper, "Institutional Policies for Responding to Allegations of Research Fraud," *IRB: A Review of Human Subjects Research* 8(4) (July/August 1986), 1, 2 (appeals procedures existed in only thirteen percent of the IRBs responding to 1982 survey directed specifically at how allegations of research fraud are handled).

19 W. J. Curran, "Medical Research on Human Subjects," (book review) *Yale Law Journal* 92 (1983): 577, 582. In my twelve months of experience as a member of the National Institutes of Neurological Diseases and Strokes' IRB at the NIH Clinical Center, we have repeatedly approved protocols subject to suggested revisions or turned them down with a request for revision and resubmission, but we have not seen a protocol in need of outright disapproval without even the option of resubmission.

20 Pub. L. No. 93-348, 88 Stat. 342 (12 July 1974).

21 Faden and Beauchamp, *A History and Theory of Informed Consent*, 217.

22 For example, TX. Rev. Civ. Stat. Ann. art. 4447d § 3 (Vernon 1976) (no indication that IRBs are included but statutory language is very broad).

23 For example, in the unreported case of *Bailey v. Mandel*, No. 74-110 (D.C. MD 1974), the American Civil Liberties Union's National Prison Project filed suit against twenty-one defendants including IRB members involved in

experiments that were done on prisoners, claiming the prisoners were living in conditions that made their consent invalid. W. W. Woodward, "An Investigator/ Defendant Corrects the Record," *IRB: A Review of Human Subject Research* 1 (4) (August/September 1979): 10; and L. M. Bordas, "Tort Liability of Institutional Review Boards," *West Virginia Law Review* 87 (Spring 1984): 141, n. 32. Aspects of the case that involved the IRB and its chairman were dismissed early on in the case. *Ibid*. Since 1979 there have been a few cases brought against IRBs, but as of October 1990 neither the office of Protection from Research Risks nor Dr. Robert Levine, an expert on IRBs at Yale University Medical School, are aware of any judgments against an IRB or its members.

24 331 N.W.2d 870 (IA 1983).

25 Bordas, "Tort Liability of Institutional Review Boards," 141, n. 32. The case was decided based on whether the records of a potential marrow donor were within the public domain without ever addressing the question of whether the IRB had acted negligently. *Head v. Colloton*, 331 N.W.2d 870 (IA 1983).

26 Department of Health and Human Services, *Code of Federal Regulations* 45 (Washington, DC: U.S. Government Printing Office, 1989), § 46.111; Food and Drug Administration, *Code of Federal Regulations* 21 (Washington, DC: U.S. Government Printing Office, 1989), § 56.111.

27 Department of Health and Human Services, *Code of Federal Regulations* 45 (Washington, DC: U.S. Government Printing Office, 1989), §§ 46.116-46.117; Food and Drug Administration, *Code of Federal Regulations* 21 (Washington, DC: U.S. Government Printing Office, 1989), § 50. Consider, for example, how adequate informed consent may have obviated some of the problems litigated in the *Baby M* case. M. Hornblower, "Baby M: Battle of 'Class and Gender'," *Washington Post* (17 February 1987): A1, A4, col. 1 (arguing that perhaps Marybeth Whitehead, the surrogate mother in the *Baby M* case, did not give informed consent).

28 Department of Health and Human Services, *Code of Federal Regulations* 45 (Washington, DC: U.S. Government Printing Office, 1989), § 46.107; Food and Drug Administration, *Code of Federal Regulations* 21 (Washington, DC: U.S. Government Printing Office, 1989), § 56.107. But see note 10 of this chapter (describing potential changes in regulation of IRB composition).

29 One example of an effort to establish mandatory guidelines for ethics committees is the Maryland state law requiring hospitals to have ethics committees. MD Health-General Code Ann. §§19-370 to 19-374 (1990) (effective 1 July 1987). See also note 39 of chapter 9 (text of relevant part of Maryland law).

30 See generally, Tribe, *American Constitutional Law*, 247-50 (discussing federal authority derived from spending power).

31 J. E. Nowak, R. D. Rotunda, and J. N. Young, *Constitutional Law*, 2d. ed. (St. Paul, MN: West Publishing Co., 1983), 121-131 (describing sources of national authority).

32 DHHS IRB regulations clearly get their authority from the federal

spending power because they apply only to research funded by DHHS. Department of Health and Human Services, *Code of Federal Regulations* 45 (Washington, DC: U.S. Government Printing Office, 1989), § 46. FDA regulation of IRBs is based on the authority of the Federal Food, Drug, and Cosmetic Act of 1938, which is based on the national authority to regulate interstate commerce. Food and Drug Administration, *Code of Federal Regulations* 21 (Washington, DC: U.S. Government Printing Office, 1989), § 56 (reference to act); Federal Food, Drug, and Cosmetic act, 21 U.S.C. §§ 321-392 (1938) (prohibited conduct specified by act all involve interstate commerce).

33   See MD Health-Gen. Code Ann. §§ 19-370 to 374 (1990).

34   Veatch, "Courts, Committees, and Caring."

35   The Maryland Bar Association is considering the possibility of suggesting to the Maryland legislature that bioethics committee decisions be binding in cases involving incompetent patients who have left no advance directives and have no family members to look after their care. Conversation with D. Hoffmann, Assistant Professor of Law, and Healthcare at the University of Maryland School of Law on 2 August 1990. Although this measure may not have the consequence of taking authority out of the hands of patients and their families or surrogates, it certainly does take the decision-making authority out of the hands of the physicians.

Chapter 9

1   The Joint Commission on Accreditation of Healthcare Organizations, which until recently was called the Joint Commission on Accreditation of Hospitals (JCAH), was organized and founded in 1951 by the American College of Surgeons, the American College of Physicians, the American Hospital Association, the American Medical Association, and the Canadian Medical Association. The Canadian Medical Association discontinued its participation in 1959 when Canada created its own program for accrediting hospitals. W. Wadlington, J. R. Waltz, and R. B. Dworkin, *Cases and Materials on Law and Medicine* (Mineola, New York: Foundation Press, 1980), 203.

From its inception, the goal of the Joint Commission has been to improve health care by setting standards that member institutions must follow to be accredited. Each year the Joint Commission publishes an accreditation manual for various types of medical institutions, setting out its minimum requirements and other aspirational standards.

2   42 U.S.C. § 1320c (1976).

3   Joint Commission, *The Joint Commission 1990 AMH: Accreditation Manual for Hospitals* (Chicago: Joint Commission, 1989), §§ MS. 1.2.3.1.5, MS.3.5.2.1.5, MS.3.7., MS.5.4. [hereinafter Joint Commission, *Accreditation Manual*].

4   The Joint Commission requires that each of a hospital's departments

perform quality review. Joint Commission, *Accreditation Manual* § MS.3.7. Hence, the committees that perform peer review often take on the name of their departments, for example, "Surgical Review Committee," "Tissue Review Committee," "Drug Usage Review Committee," "Records Review Committee," etc.

5   *Ibid.*

6   Joint Commission on Accreditation of Hospitals, *JCAH 1982, AMH: Accreditation Manual* (Chicago: Joint Commission on Accreditation of Hospitals, 1982), 106.

7   "Surgical case review is performed monthly by those departments/services performing surgical procedures or by a medical staff committee to help assure that surgery performed in the hospital is justified and of high quality." Joint Commission, *Accreditation Manual*, § MS.6.1.2.1.

8   A combination of departments and services are responsible for establishing a medical record review function that "assures that each medical record, or a representative sample of records, reflects the diagnosis, results of diagnostic tests, therapy rendered, condition and in-hospital progress of a patient, and condition of the patient at discharge." *Ibid.*, § MS.6.1.4.2.2.

9   "The executive committee is responsible for making recommendations directly to the governing body for its approval. Such recommendations pertain to... [t]he mechanism used to review credentials and to delineate individual clinical privileges. The organization of the quality assurance activities of the medical staff as well as the mechanism used to conduct, evaluate, and revise such activities. The mechanism by which membership on the medical staff may be terminated . . ." *Ibid.*, MS.3.5.

10   Roundtree, "The Anguish of Peer Review," *Journal of the Medical Association of Georgia* 67 (April 1978): 287.

11   D. W. Jorstad, "The Legal Liability of Medical Peer Review Participants for Revocation of Hospital Staff Privileges," *Drake Law Review* 28 (1978-79) L, 697-716.

12   MA Ann. Laws Ch. 111, § 203(a) (Law. Co-op. 1988 Supp.).

13   AZ Rev. Stat. Ann. § 36-2404 (1988).

14   ME Rev. Stat. Ann. tit. 24 § 2506 (1988 Supp.).

15   IA Code § 54-934 (1988).

16   Jorstad, "The Legal Liability of Medical Peer Review Participants for Revocation of Hospital Staff Privileges," 694.

17   For example, MN Stat. § 145.63 (West 1989).

18   *Ibid.*

19   For example, MD Code Health-Occupations Ann. § 14-601 (f) (1986).

20   See generally, Keeton, Dobbs, Keeton, and Owen, *Prosser and Keeton on the Law of Torts*, 1032-33, 1043-71 (describing forms of sovereign and charitable immunities).

21   For example, CA Evid. Code § 1157 (1966 and 1990 Supp.)

22 For example, CA Evid. Code § 1157 (1966 and 1990 Supp.) provides immunity from discovery for all medical staff committee proceedings, while CA Civ. Code § 43.7(b) (1982 and 1990 Supp.) only provides immunity from civil liability if the committee is composed primarily of health-care professionals. IL Ann. Stat. ch. 110 § 8-2101 (Smith-Hurd 1984 and 1989 Supp.) grants committee proceedings immunity from discovery but does not grant committee members immunity from liability. IL Ann. Stat. ch. 110 § 8-2103 (Smith-Hurd 1984) grants immunity from liability but only for those who furnish information to medical staff committees.

23 Pub. L. No. 99-660 *U.S. Code Cong. & Admin. News* (99 Stat.) *U.S. Code*, Vol. 42, secs. 11101-52 (1986). (effective as of 14 November 1986 for federal laws; effective as of 14 October 1989 for state laws unless states chose to push up that date or exempt themselves from the act).

24 *Ibid.*, § 402.

25 *Ibid.*, §§ 411-412.

26 *Ibid.*, § 427 (b).

27 *Ibid.*, § 411.

28 *Ibid.*

29 *Ibid.*

30 See notes 16-19 of this chapter and accompanying text (states with limits on immunity).

31 Pub. L. No. 99-660, § 412, *U.S. Code Cong. & Admin. News* (99 Stat.) (Nov. 14, 1986).

32 *Ibid.*

33 *Ibid.*, §§ 422-427.

34 *Ibid.*, § 423.

35 *Ibid.*, § 422.

36 *Ibid.*, § 427.

37 *Ibid.*, § 423, 427(b).

38 See notes 7-9 of this chapter and accompanying text (description of peer review committee functions).

39 It should be noted, however, that the Maryland law mandating bioethics committees also provides for limited liability and disclosure.

(c) Liability for advice.--An advisory committee [Maryland name for bioethics committee] or a member of an advisory committee who gives advice in good faith may not be held liable in court for the advice given.

(d) Confidentiality.--(1) The proceedings and deliberations of an advisory committee are confidential as provided in § 14.601 of the Health Occupations Article [providing immunity from disclosure for peer review committees].

MD Health-Gen. Code Ann. §§ 19-374(c) (1990). The only restriction is that the advice be given in good faith. This law makes no distinction between criminal and civil cases, nor does it require that advice be given in the context of the

committee's assigned duties. For laws that do make such distinctions, see HI Rev. Stat. § 663-1.7 (1989 Supp.); and MT Code Ann. § 37-2-1 (1989).
40 *Ibid.*

Chapter 10

1 Department of Health and Human Services, "Nondiscrimination on the Basis of Handicap; Procedures and Guidelines Relating to Health Care for Handicapped Infants," *Federal Register* 49 (12 January 1984): 1622-1654.
2 U.S., 110 S. Ct. 2841 (1990).
3 U.S., 109 S. Ct. 3040 (1989).
4 E. Friedman, "New Directions for the JCAH?" *Hospitals* (16 November 1985): 120 (the quotation is from interviewee D. S. O'Leary, then President-Elect of the JCAH) (emphasis added).
5 MD Health-Gen. Code Ann. §§ 19-370 to 374 (1990).
6 The Secretary of the Maryland Department of Health and Human Hygiene is responsible for licensing, sanctioning, and revoking of licensure for hospitals. MD Health-General Code Ann. §§ 19-306, 19-308, 19-327 (1990). Maryland also has a board of medical professionals, the State Advisory Board on Hospitals, that advises the Secretary of the Department of Health and Human Hygiene on the approval or denial of licensure applications. *Ibid.*, § 19-306.
7 Murphy, "Malpractice Allegation Is Added to Bouvia's Lawsuit," *Los Angeles Times*, 8 October 1986, p. 3, part 2, col. 1. This suit is *not* the one where the California Appeals Court granted Bouvia the right to refuse tube feeding. *Elizabeth Bouvia v. Superior Court (Glenchur)*, 225 CA App. 3d 1127 (CA 1986). It is a separate suit for damages filed in the Los Angeles Superior Court. There were two suits for damages filed by Elizabeth Bouvia in the Los Angeles County Superior Cout. It is unclear which one included her action against the High Desert Hospital bioethics committee, but both suits were dismissed in November 1989. *Bouvia v. Gates, et al.*, Civil Case No. C596997 (Los Angeles Superior Court, dismissed 1 November 1989); *Bouvia v. Fleischman, et al.*, Civil Case No. C583828 (Los Angeles County Superior Court, dismissed 12 November 1989).
8 Murphy, "Malpractice Allegation Is Added to Bouvia's Lawsuit," (emphasis added).
9 See note 6 for this chapter.
10 D. W. Jorstad, "The Legal Liability of Medical Peer Review Participants for Revocation of Hospital Staff Privileges," *Drake Law Review* 28 (1978-79) L, 697-716.
11 Keeton, Dobbs, Keeton, and Owen, *Prosser and Keeton on the Law of Torts*, 185-93.
12 *Ibid.*
13 *Ibid.*

14 Henn, and Alexander, *Laws of Corporations and Other Business Enterprises*, §§ 234, 235 and 1986 Supp. at 21.

15 For example, PA Bus. Corp. Law § 408(b) (as amended in 1983) (law includes interest other than those of corporation among directors' fiduciary duties).

16 *Ibid.*, § 218.

17 K.B. Davis, "Judicial Review of Fiduciary Decisionmaking: Some Theoretical Perspectives" *Northwestern University Law Review* 80 (1985) (discussing dual origin [private ordering and law] of fiduciary principles).

18 Keeton, Dobbs, Keeton, and Owen, *Prosser and Keeton on the Law of Torts*, 164-165.

19 *Ibid.*, 54-65.

20 For example, a bioethics committee could be guilty of intentional or reckless infliction of emotional distress if, after in vitro fertilization had taken place, but before implantation, the bioethics committee had a change of heart and requested that the pre-embryo be destroyed without consulting the physician or the patients who had come for infertility treatment. See *Del Zio v. The Presbyterian Hospital*, 74 NY Civ. Ct. 3588 (1978) (hospital was found liable for intentional infliction of emotional distress for destroying fertilized ova without notifying attending physician).

21 Keeton, Dobbs, Keeton, and Owen, *Prosser and Keeton on the Law of Torts*, 773-74.

22 The term "civil rights" is used broadly to include any individual or minority rights the government protects against its own actions or those of private individuals.

23 See generally, Abraham, *Freedom and the Court, Civil Rights and Liberties in the United States* (discussing various types of civil rights protections); Tribe, *American Constitutional Law*, 256-275 (same).

24 *Ibid.*

25 The Civil Rights Commission report was released on 22 September 1989. S. Fry-Revere, "Legal Trends in Bioethics," *The Journal of Clinical Ethics* (Summer 1990): 162-63.

26 S. H. Dadish, S. J. Schulhofer, and M. G. Paulsen, *Criminal Law and Its Processes: Cases and Materials*, 4th ed. (Boston: Little, Brown and Co., 1983), 643-720.

27 *Ibid.*

28 *United States v. Alvarez*, 610 F.2d (5th Cir. 1980).

BIBLIOGRAPHY

Principal Sources

Books

Abraham, Henry J. *Freedom and the Court: Civil Rights and Liberties in the United States*, 4th ed. New York: Oxford University Press, 1982.

Bonnicksen, Andrea L. *In Vitro Fertilization: Policy Building from Laboratories to Legislatures*. New York: Columbia University Press, 1989.

Campion, Frank D. *The AMA and U.S. Health Policy Since 1940*. Chicago: Chicago Review Press, 1984.

Cranford, Ronald E., and Edward Doudera. *Institutional Ethics Committees and Health Care Decision Making*. Ann Arbor, Michigan: Health Administration Press, 1984.

Davis, Nathan Smith. *History of the American Medical Association from Its Organization up to January 1855.* Edited by Samuel Worcester Butler. Philadephia: Lippincott, Grambo and Co., 1855.

Derbyshire, Robert Cushing. *Medical Licensure and Discipline in the United States.* Baltimore: Johns Hopkins Press, 1969.

Dworkin, Ronald. *Law's Empire*. Cambridge, Massachussetts: Belknap Press, 1986.

Engelhardt, Jr., H. Tristram. *The Foundations of Bioethics.* New York: Oxford University Press, 1986.

Faden, Ruth R., and Tom L. Beauchamp. *A History and Theory of Informed Consent.* New York: Oxford University Press, 1986.

Fletcher, John C., Norman Quist, and Albert R. Jonsen, eds. *Ethics Consultation in Health Care*. Ann Arbor, Michigan: Health Administration Press, 1989.

Friedman, Milton. *Capitalism and Freedom*. Chicago: University of Chicago Press, 1962.

Gosfield, Alice G., ed. *1989 Health Law Handbook*. New York: Clark Boardman Co., Ltd., 1989.

Grad, Frank P., and Noelia Marti. *Physicians' Licensure and Discipline: The Legal and Professional Regulation of Medical Practice*. Dobbs Ferry, New York: Oceana, Publications, Inc., 1979.

Henn, Harry G., and John R. Alexander. *Laws of Corporations and Other Business Enterprises*, 3d ed. St. Paul, Minnesota: West Publishing Co., 1983 and 1986 Supplement.

Hosford, Bowen. *Bioethics Committees: The Health Care Provider's Guide*. Rockville, Maryland: Aspen Systems Corporation, 1986.

Katz, Jay. *Experimentation with Human Beings: The Authority of the Investigator, Subject, Professions and State in the Human Experimentation Process*. New York: Russel Sage Foundation, 1972.

Keeton, W., D. Dobbs, R. Keeton, and D. Owen. *Prosser and Keeton on the Law of Torts*. 5th ed. St. Paul, Minnesota: West Publishing Co., 1984.

National Science Foundation. *Self-Regulation in the Professions: Accounting, Law, Medicine*. Principal Investigator Hedvah L. Shuchman. Glastonbury, Connecticut: Futures Group, July 1981.

Rawls, John. *A Theory of Justice*. Cambridge, Massachussetts: Harvard University Press, 1971.

Tribe, Lawrence H. *American Constitutional Law*. Mineola, New York: Foundation Press, 1978.

Wadlington, Walter, Jon R. Waltz, and Roger B. Dworkin. *Cases and Materials on Law and Medicine*. Mineola, New York: Foundation Press, 1980.

Weinstein, Bruce, ed. *Ethics in the Hospital Setting*. Morgantown, West Virginia: West Virginia University Press, 1985.

Essays

Annas, George J. "Legal Aspects of Ethics Committees." In *Institutional Ethics Committees and Health Care Decision Making,* edited by Ronald E. Cranford and A. Edward Doudera, 51-59. Ann Arbor, Michigan: Health Administration Press, 1984.

Capron, Alexander M. "Legal Perspectives on Institutional Ethics Committees." In *Ethics in the Hospital Setting,* edited by Bruce D. Weinstein, 66-84. Morgantown, West Virginia: West Virginia University Press, 1985.

Evans, Marien E. "Legal Background of the IRB." *In Human Subjects Research: A Handbook for Institutional Review Boards,* edited by Robert A. Greenwald, Mary Kay Ryan, and James E. Mulvihill, 19-28. New York: Plenum Press, 1982.

Reich, Warren T. ed. *The Encyclopedia of Bioethics,* Vol. 3. New York: The Free Press, 1978. S.v. II-Organized Medicine, by James G. Burrow.

Self, Donnie J., and Joy D. Skeel. "Legal Liability and Clinical Ethics Consultations: Practical and Philosophical Considerations." In *Medical Ethics: A Guide for Health Professionals,* edited by John F. Monagle and David C. Thomasma. Rockville, Maryland: Aspen Publishers, Inc., 1988.

Thomasma, David C., and John F. Monagle. "Hospital Ethics Committees: Roles, Membership, and Structure." In *Medical Ethics: A Guide for Health Professionals*, edited by John E. Monagle and David C. Thomasma. Rockville, Maryland: Aspen Publishers, Inc., 1988.

Welt, Louis G. "Reflections on the Problems of Human Experimentation." In *Experimentation with Human Beings: The Authority of the Investigator, Subject, Professions and State in the Human Experimentation Process.* by Jay Katz. New York: Russell Sage Foundation, 1972.

Wicclair, Mark R. "The Distinction Between Medical and Ethical Decisions." In *Ethics in the Hospital Setting*, edited by Bruce Weinstein. Morgantown, West Virginia: West Virginia University Press, 1985.

Youngner, Stuart J., David L. Jackson, Claudia Coulton, Barbara W. Juknialis, and Era Smith. "A National Survey of Hospital Ethics Committees." In *Deciding to Forego Life-Sustaining Treatment: Ethical, Medical and Legal Issues in Treatment Decisions*, by President's Commission for the Study of Ethical Problems in Medicine and Biomedical and Behavioral Research. Washington DC: U.S. Government Printing Office, 1983.

Journal Articles

Avard, D., G. Griener, and J. Langstaff. "Hospital Ethics Committees: Survey Reveals Characteristics." *Dimensions in Health Service* 62 (February 1985): 24-26.

Breaden, Dale G., and Bryant L. Balusha. "Official 1985 Federation Summary of Reported Disciplinary Actions." *Federation Bulletin* (October 1986): 300.

Butler, Randall E. "Hospital Peer Review Committees: Privileges of Confidentiality and Immunity." *South Texas Law Journal* 23 (1) (1982): 45-69.

Craig-Clark, Dianne. "Bouvia Names Ethics Committee Members in Malpractice Suit." *Medical Ethics Advisor* 2 (December 1986): 153-55.

Davis, Kenneth B. "Judicial Review of Fiduciary Decisionmaking: Some Theoretical Perspectives." *Northwestern University Law Review* 80 (1985): 1-99.

Dine, Deborah, "Ethics Panels Multiplying to Grapple with Tough Issues." *Modern Healthcare* (14 October 1988): 22-30.

Feinstein, Richard J. "Special Report: The Ethics of Professional Regulation." *New England Journal of Medicine* 312 (12) (21 March 1985): 801-04.

Fost, Norman, and Ronald E. Cranford. "Hospital Ethics Committees: Administrative Aspects." *Journal of the American Medical Association* 235 (18) (10 May 1985): 2687-92.

Holder, Angela R. "Liability and the IRB Member: The Legal Aspects." *IRB: A Review of Human Subjects Research* 1 (3) (May 1979): 7-8.

Kadish, Sanford H. "Methodology and Criteria in Due Process Adjudication-- A Survey and Criticism." *Yale Law Journal* 66 (1956-1957): 319-363.

King, Lester S. "The Founding of the American Medical Association. *Journal of the American Medical Association* 248 (8 October 1982): 149-1752.

Latin, Howard A. "Problem-Solving Behavior and Theories of Tort Liability." *California Law Review* 73 (1985): 677-83.

Levine, Carol. "Hospital Ethics Committees: A Guarded Prognosis." *Hastings Center Report* 7 (June 1977): 25, 27.

Merritt, Andrew L. "The Tort Liability of Hospital Ethics Committees." *Southern California Law Review* 60 (1987): 1239-97.

Postell, Claudia J. "Clergy Malpractice: An Emerging Field of Law." *Trial* 21 (December 1985): 91-93.

Rosner, Fred. "Hospital Medical Ethics Committees: A Review of Their Development." *Journal of the American Medical Association* 253 (10 May 1985): 2693, 2695.

Veatch, Robert M. "Courts, Committees, and Caring." *American Medical News* 23 (23 May 1980): Impact/1 - Impact 2 + .

Walters, LeRoy. "Commissions and Bioethics." *Journal of Medicine and Philosophy* 14 (4) (August 1989): 363-368.

Weir, Robert F. "Pediatric Ethics Committees: Ethical Advisers or Legal Watchdogs?" *Law, Medicine & Health Care* 15 (3) (Fall 1987): 99-109.

Wolf, Susan M. "Ethics Committees in the Courts." *Hastings Center Report* 16 (3) (June 1986): 12-15.

Newspaper and Newsletter Articles

Murphy, Kim. "Malpractice Allegation Is Added to Bouvia's Lawsuit." *Los Angeles Times*, 8 October 1986, p. 3, Part 2, Col. 1.

"Suing Clergymen for Malpractice." *Time,* 12 January 1981, p. 75.

Official Documents and Regulations

American Medical Association. "Report QQ" (AMA Initiative on Quality of Medical Care and Professional Self-Regulation.) In *Journal of the American Medical Association* 256 (8) (22/29 August 1986): 1036-37.

American Medical Association. *Physician Characteristics and Distribution in the US*. Chicago: American Medical Association, 1986.

Joint Commission for Accreditation of Healthcare Organizations. *Joint Commission 1990 AMH: Accreditation Manual for Hospitals*. Chicago: Joint Commission on Accreditation of Healthcare Organizations, 1989.

National Commission for the Protection of Human Subjects of Biomedical and Behavioral Research. *Report and Recommendations: Institutional Review*

Boards. Washington, DC: U.S. Printing Office, DHEW Publication No. (OS) 78-0008, 1978.

National Institutes of Health. "Group Consideration for Clinical Research Procedures Deviating from Accepted Medical Practice or Involving Unusual Hazard," (17 November 1953). In *Ethics and Regulation of Clinical Research*, edited by Robert Levine. Baltimore: Urban and Schwarzenberg, 1981.

U.S. Department of Health and Human Services. *Code of Federal Regulations*. Title 45, sec. 46. Washington, D.C.: US Government Printing Office, 1989.

U.S. Department of Health and Human Services. "Final Regulations Amending Basic HHS Policy for the Protection of Human Research Subjects." *Federal Register* 46 (26 January 1981): 8366-8401.

U.S. Department of Health and Human Services. "Nondiscrimination on the Basis of Handicap; Procedures and Guidelines Relating to Health Care for Handicapped Infants; Final Rule." *Federal Register* 49 (16 January 1984): 1621-1654.

U.S. Food and Drug Administration, *Code of Federal Regulations*. Title 21, secs. 50, 56. Washington, DC: US Government Printing Office, 1989.

Unpublished Papers and Documents

Areen, Judith. "Legal Implications of Ethics Consultation." A presentation at a conference co-sponsored by the National Institutes of Health and the University of California at San Francisco, 7-8 October 1985.

Areen, Judith. "Analysis of Maryland Law Patient Care Advisory Committees 19-370-74 (Health-General). 1986.

Fletcher, John C. "Standards for Evaluation of Ethics Consultations." A presentation at a conference co-sponsored by the National Institutes of Health and the University of California at San Francisco, 7-8 October 1985. Revised version published in Fletcher, John C., Norman Quist, and Albert R. Jonsen, eds. *Ethics Consultation in Health Care*. Ann Arbor, Michigan: Health Administration Press, 1989. 173-184.

Robertson, John A. "Clinical Medical Ethics and the Law: The Rights and Duties of Ethics Consultants." A presentation at a conference co-sponsored by the National Institutes of Health and the University of California at San Francisco, 7-8 October, 1985. Revised version published in Fletcher, John

C., Norman Quist, and Albert R. Jonsen, eds. *Ethics Consultation in Health Care*, 157-172. Ann Arbor, Michigan: Health Administration Press, 1989.

Society for Bioethics Consultation. "IRS [Internal Revenue Service]--Activities and Operational Description, Draft Articles of Incorporation (1986).

Cases

Lund v. Caple, 675 P.2d 226 (WA 1984).

McCutcheon v. The Arch Dyasis of Washington, (Mont County Cir. Ct. 1988).

Nally v. Grace Community Church of the Valley, 253 CA Rptr. 97 (1988).

Niccoli v. Thompson, 713 S.W.2d 579 (MO App. 1986).

Oliver v. Brock, 342 So.2d 1 (AL 1976).

Sullenger v. Setco Northwest, 702 P.2d 1139 (OR App 1985).

Statutes

Health Care Quality Improvement Act of 1986. 14 Nov 1986, Public Law No. 99-660, 1986 *US Code*. Vol. 42, secs. 11101-52 (1986).

Maryland Health-General Code Annotated. Secs. 19-370 to 19-374 (West 1986).

The Patient Self-Determination Act, passed as part of the *Budget Reconciliation Act of 1990*, 42 US Code sec. 1395cc(a)(1) (Medicare Provider Agreements Assuring the Implementation of a Patient's Right to Participation in and Direct Health Care Decisons Affecting the Patient).

The Social Security Act. Secs. 1151 *et seq.*, 42 US Code, sec. 1320c (1982 and 1989 Supplement).

The Social Security Amendments of 1972, US Public Law No. 92-603.

Other Sources

Books

Aquinas, Thomas. *Summa Theologica*. In *Introduction to Saint Thomas Aquinas*, edited by A. C. Pegis. New York: Random House, Inc., 1945.

American Board of Medical Specialties. *Directory of Medical Specialties: 1979-1980*, 19th ed., Vol. 1. Evanston, Illinois: Marquia Who's Who, 1979.

Anscombe, G. E. M. *Intention*. Ithaca, New York: Cornell University Press, 1969.

Aristotle. *Nichomachean Ethics*. Translated by Terence Irwin. Indianapolis, Indiana: Hackett Publishing Co., 1985.

Backus, Karen, edited by *Encyclopedia of Medical Organizations and Agencies*. Detroit, Michigan: Gale Research Inc., 1990.

Beauchamp, Tom L., and Laurence B. McCullough. *Medical Ethics: The Moral Responsibilities of Physicians*. Englewood Cliffs, New Jersey: Prentice-Hall, Inc., 1984.

Broad, C. D. *The Mind and Its Place in Nature*. London: Routledge & Kegan Paul, Ltd., 1925.

Christoffel, Tom. *Health and the Law: A Handbook for Health Professionals*. New York: The Free Press, 1982.

Dadish, Sanford H., Stephen J. Schulhfer, and Monrad G. Paulsen. *Criminal Law and Its Processes: Cases and Materials*, 4th edited by Boston: Little, Brown and Co., 1983.

Ely, John Hart. *Democracy and Distrust: a Theory of Judicial Review*. Cambridge, Massachusetts: Harvard University Press, 1980.

Emmet, Dorothy. *Rules, Rules and Relations*. London: Macmillan Co., 1966.

Ewing, A. E. *The Definition of Good*. New York: Macmillan Co., 1947.

Feinberg, Joel. *Doing and Deserving: Essays in the Theory of Responsibility*. Princeton: Princeton University Press, 1970.

Fletcher, Joseph F. *Situation Ethics: The New Morality*. Philadelphia: Westminster Press, 1966.

Fromer, Margot J. *Ethical Issues in Health Care*. St. Louis: Mosby Co., 1981.

Glover, Jonathan. *Responsibility*. New York: Humanities Press, 1970.

Goodin, Robert E. *Political Theory & Public Policy*. Chicago: University of Chicago Press, 1982.

Goodin, Robert E. *Manipulatory Politics*. New Haven: Yale University Press, 1980.

Hart, H. L. A. *The Concept of Law*. Oxford: Clarendon Press; 1961.

Hart, H.L.A. *Punishment and Responsibility: Essays in the Philosophy of Law*. Oxford: Oxford University Press, 1967. 186-209, 211-30

Hart, H.L.A., and A. M. Honor. *Causation in the Law*. Oxford: Oxford University Press, 1959.

Hobbes. *Leviathan*. Edited by C. B. Macpherson. Middlesex: Penguin Books, 1968.

Hospers, John. *Human Conduct*. New York: Harcourt, Brace & World, 1961.

Kant, Immanuel. *Foundations of the Metaphysics of Morals*. Translated by L. W. Beck. Indianapolis: Bobbs-Merrill Comp., Inc., 1959.

Kass, Leon R. *Toward a More Natural Science*. New York: Free Press, 1985.

Levine, Robert J. *Ethics and Regulation of Clinical Research*. Baltimore: Urban & Schwarzenberg, 1981.

Lieberman, Jethro K. *The Tyranny of the Experts*. New York: Walker and Company, 1970.

Locke, John. *Two Treatises of Government*. Introduction and notes by Peter Laslett. Cambridge: Cambridge University Press, 1960.

MacPherson, C. B. *Democratic Theory: Essays in Retrieval*. Oxford: Clarendon Press, 1973.

Maloney, Dennis M. *Protection of Human Research Subjects: A Practical Guide to Federal Laws and Regulations*. New York: Plenum Press, 1984.

Mill, John Stuart. *On Liberty*. In *John Stuart Mill: A Selection of His Works*, edited by J. M. Robson. Indianapolis: The Bobbs-Merrill Comp., Inc., 1966.

Nowak, John E., Ronald D. Rotunda, and J. Nelson Young *Constitutional Law,* 2d. edited by St. Paul, Minnesota: West Publishing Co., 1983.

Nozick, Robert. *Philosophical Explanations.* Cambridge, Massachusetts: Belknap Press of Harvard University Press, 1981.

Pitkin, Hanna Fenichel. *The Concept of Representation.* Berkeley: University of California Press, 1967.

Plato, *The Republic.* In *The Dialogues of Plato.* Vol. 3, translated by Ernest Barker. London: Oxford University Press, 1977.

Semin, G. R., and A. S. R. Manstead. *The Accountability of Conduct.* London: Academic Press, 1983.

Souter, Alexander. *Texts and Studies.* Vol. 9, *Pelagius' Expositions of the 13 Epistles of St. Paul.* Cambridge: Cambridge University Press, 1926.

Stace, Walter T. *Religion and the Modern Mind.* New York: Harper & Row Publishers, Inc., 1952.

Szasz, Thomas. *Law, Liberty and Psychiatry.* New York: Macmillan Co., 1963.

Taylor, Richard. *Metaphysics*, 2d. edited by Englewood Cliffs, New Jersey: Prentice-Hall, Inc., 1974.

Veatch, Robert M. *A Theory of Medical Ethics.* New York: Basic Books, Inc., 1981.

Walzer, Michael. *Spheres of Justice.* New York: Basic Books, 1983.

Webster's New World Dictionary of the American Language, 2nd ed.

Wolfram, Charles W. *Modern Legal Ethics.* St. Paul, Minnesota: West Publishing Co., 1986.

Essays

Agich, George J. "The Concept of Responsibility in Medicine." In *Responsibility in Health Care*, edited by George J. Agich. 53-64. Dordrecht, Holland: D. Reidel Publishing Company, 1982.

Feinberg, Joel. "On Justifying Legal Punishment." In *Responsibility*, edited by Carl J. Friedrich. 152-170. New York: Liberal Arts Press, Inc., 1960. 152-170.

Feinberg, Joel. "Punishment." In *Philosophy of Law*, 3d ed., edited by Joel Feinberg and Hyman Gross. 587-602. Belmont, California: Wadsworth Publishing Co., 1986.

Feinberg, Joel. "Responsibility." In *Philosophy of Law,* 3d ed., edited by Joel Feinberg and Hyman Gross. 467-73. Belmont, California: Wadsworth Publishing Co., 1986.

Feinberg, Joel. "Sua Culpa." In *Philosophy of Law*, 3d ed., edited by Joel Feinberg and Hyman Gross. 512-27. Belmont, California: Wadsworth Publishing Co., 1986.

Fletcher, John C., and Maxwell Boverman. "Evolution of the Role of an Applied Bioethicist in a Research Hospital." In *Research Ethics*, edited by Kare Berg and Knut E. Tranoy. 131-158. New York: Alan R. Liss Co., 1983.

Freund, Ludwig. "Responsibility--Definitions, Distinctions, and Applications in Various Contexts." In *Responsibility*, edited by Carl J. Friedrich, 28-42. New York: Liberal Arts Press, Inc., 1960.

Friedrich, Carl J. " The Dilemma of Administrative Responsibility." In *Responsibility*, edited by Carl J. Friedrich. 152-170. 189-202. New York: Liberal Arts Press, Inc., 1960.

Friedson, Eliot. *The Profession of Medicine: A Study of the Sociology of Applied Knowledge.* Chicago: University of Chicago Press, 1970.

Guido, Doris Jordan. "Hospital Ethics Committees: Potential Mediators of Educational and Policy Change." In *Dissertation Abstracts International*. Vol. 43, p. 3529. Michigan: University Microfilms International, 1983.

Knight, F. H. "Political Responsibility in a Democracy." In *Responsibility*, edited by Carl J. Friedrich. 171-188. New York: Liberal Arts Press, Inc., 1960.

Kohrman, Arthur F. "Comments on 'The Concept of Responsibility in Medicine.' " In *Responsibility in Health Care*, edited by George J. Agich. 75-82. Dordrecht, Holland: D. Reidel Publishing Company, 1982.

Mackie, J. L. "The Grounds of Responsibility." In *Law, Morality, and Society: Essays in Honour of H. L. A. Hart,* edited by P. M. S. Hacker and J. Raz, 175-188. Oxford: Clarendon Press, 1977.

Macklin, Ruth. "Consultative Roles and Responsibilities." In *Institutional Ethics Committees and Health Care Decision Making,* edited by Ronald E. Cranford and A. Edward Doudera. 157-168. Ann Arbor, Michigan: Health Administration Press, 1984.

Miller, Bruce L. "Responsibility and Public Policy in Health Care: Commentary on Essays by Williams and Rich." In *Responsibility in Health Care,* edited by George J. Agich, 261-76. Dordrecht, Holland: D. Reidel Publishing Company, 1982.

Pennock, J. Roland. "The Problem of Responsibility." In *Responsibility*, edited by Carl J. Friedrich. 3-27. New York: Liberal Arts Press, Inc., 1960.

Wootton, Barbara. "Eliminating Responsibility." In *Philosophy of Law*, 3d ed., edited by Joel Feinberg and Hyman Gross. 543-57. Belmont, California: Wadsworth Publishing Co., 1986.

Journal Articles

American Hospital Association. "AMA Stymies Patient 'Bill of Rights.'" *Hospital Ethics* 6 (1) (January/February 1990): 4.

Aroskar, Mila A. "Establishing Limits to Professional Autonomy: Whose Responsibility?" *Nursing Law & Ethics* 1 (5) (May 1980): 1-2.

Barnett, Randy E. "Restitution: A New Paradigm of Criminal Justice." *Ethics* 87 (4) (July 1977): 279-301.

Barry, Robert L. "Infant Care Review Committees: Their Moral Responsibilities." *Linacre Quarterly* 52 (4) (November 1985): 361-74.

Bennett, Daniel. "Action, Reason, and Purpose." *Journal of Philosophy* 62 (4) (18 February 1965): 85-95.

Blumstein, James F. "Responsibility and Accountability in Provider-Patient Relationships." *Circulation* 66 Supplement III (1982): III-91-99.

"Board Certification and Physicians' Income." *Pro Forum* 1 (1) (June 1978): 4.

Bordas, Linda M. "Tort Liability of Institutional Review Boards." *West Virginia Law Review* 87 (Spring 1984): 137-164.

Brooks, Lee W. "Intentional Infliction of Emotional Distress by Spiritual Counselors: Can Outrageous Conduct Be Free Exercise?" *Michigan Law Review* 84 (May 1986): 1296-1325.

Browne, Alister. "Ethics Committees for What?" Editorial. *Canadian Medical Association Journal* 36 (11) (1 June 1987): 1149-1151.

Burt, Robert. "The Limits of Law in Regulating Health Care Decisions." *Hastings Center Report* 7 (6) (December 1977): 29-32.

Caplan, Arthur L. "Can Applied Ethics be Effective in Health Care and Should It Strive to Be?" *Ethics* 93 (2) (January 1983): 311-19.

Capron, Alexander Morgan. "Bioethics on the Congressional Agenda." *Hastings Center Report*. 19 (2) (March/April 1989): 22-23.

Churchill, Larry R. "The Ethicist in Professional Education." *Hastings Center Report* 8 (6) (December 1978):13-15.

Churchill, Larry R. "Moralist, Technician, Sophist, Teacher/Learner: Reflections on the Ethicist in the Clinical Setting." *Theoretical Medicine* 7 (1) (February 1986): 3-12.

Churchill, Larry R., and Alan W. Cross. "The Professionalization of Ethics: Some Implications for Accountability in Medicine." *Soundings* 60 (1) (Spring 1977): 40-43.

Cohen, Cynthia B. "Interdisciplinary Consultation on the Care of the Critically Ill and Dying: The Role of One Hospital Ethics Committee." *Critical Care Medicine* 10 (11) (November 1982): 776-84.

Conway, David A. "Capital Punishment and Deterrence: Some Consideration in Dialogue Form." *Philosophy & Public Affairs* 3 (4) (Summer, 1974): 431-443.

Cranford, Ronald E., and Edward Doudera. "The Emergence of Institutional Ethics Committees." *Law, Medicine & Health Care* (February 1984): 13-20.

Cranford, David A., and Evelyn J. Van Allen. "The Implications and Applications of Institutional Ethics Committees." *Bulletin of the American College of Surgeons* 70 (6) (June 1985): 19-24.

Cranford, David A., F. Allen Hester, and Barbara Ziegler Ashley. "Institutional Ethics Committees: Issues of Confidentiality and Immunity." *Law, Medicine & Health Care* 13 (2) (April 1985): 52-60.

Curran, William J. "Medical Research on Human Subjects." Book Review. *Yale Law Journal* 92 (1983): 577-584.

Dawson, Anthony. "The Accountability of Doctor to Doctor." *Lancet* (10 August 1985): 323-24.

Feinstein, Richard J. "Special Report: The Ethics of Professional Regulation." *New England Journal of Medicine* 13 (2) (21 March 1985): 801.

Ferguson, Cherry G. "Medical Ethics Committees--the Decision is Yours." *Dimensions in Health Service* 61 (September 1984): 36-41.

Fletcher, John C. "Goals and Process of Ethics Consultation in Health Care." *BioLaw: A Legal and Ethical Reporter on Medicine, Health Care, and Bioengineering.* 2 (2) (November 1986): U: 907

Friedman, Emily. "New Directions for the JCAH?" *Hospitals* (16 November 1985): 68, 73.

Friedman, Emily. "Systemwide Ethics Centers Respond to Needs of Members, Others." *Health Progress* 67 (8) (October 1986): 41-45.

Fry-Revere, Sigrid. "Legal Trends in Bioethics." *The Journal of Clinical Ethics* (Summer 1990): 162-63.

Fry-Revere, Sigrid. "Legal Trends in Bioethics." *The Journal of Clinical Ethics* (Spring 1991): 72.

Gibson, Joan M., and Thomasine K. Kushner. "Will the 'Conscience of an Institution' Become Society's Servant?" *Hastings Center Report* 16 (3) (June 1986): 9-11.

Greene, Penelope J., Durch, Horwitz, and Hopper. "Institutional Policies for Responding to Allegations of Research Fraud." *IRB: A Review of Human Subjects Research* 8 (4) (July/August 1986): 1-7.

Grodin, Michael A., *et al.* "A 12-Year Audit of IRB Decisions." *Quality Review Bulletin* 12 (3) (March 1986): 82-86.

Haydon, Graham. "On Being Responsible." *Philosophical Quarterly* 28 (1978): 46-57.

Hayes, John R. "Consultation-Liaison Psychiatry and Clinical Ethics: A Model for Consultation and Teaching." *General Hospital Psychiatry* 8 (6) (November 1986): 415-18.

Hirsh, Harold L. "Physician's Legal Liability to Third Parties Who Are Not Patients." *Medical Trial Technique Quarterly* 23 (4) (Spring 1977): 388-400.

"It's Over Debbie, A Piece of My Mind." *Journal of the American Medical Association* 259 (8 January 1988): 272.

Jorstad, David W. "The Legal Liability of Medical Peer Review Participants for Revocation of Hospital Staff Privileges." *Drake Law Review* 28 (1978-79): 693-717.

Lo, Bernard. "Behind Closed Doors. Promises and Pitfalls of Ethics Committees." *New England Journal of Medicine* 317 (1) (2 July 1987): 46-50.

McCormick, Richard A. "Ethics Committees: Promise or Peril?" *Law, Medicine & Health Care* 12 (4) (September 1984): 150-55.

Morgan, Cheryl. "Confidentiality in a Case-Report." Letter. *Lancet* 1 (8429) (16 March 1985): 644.

Morris, Herbert. "Person and Punishment." *Monist* 52 (4) (October 1968): 475-501.

Murphy, F. Kevin, and H. Bruce Dull. "Identification of Patients." Letter. *Annals of Internal Medicine* 79 (6) (December 1973): 907.

Newton, Lisa. "A Framework for Responsible Medicine." *Journal of Medicine and Philosophy* 4 (1) (March 1979): 57-69.

Noble, Cheryl N. "Ethics and Experts: Have Philosophers Substituted Moral Reasoning for Moral Wisdom?" *Hastings Center Report* 12 (3) (June 1982): 7-9.

Pattullo, E. L. "Institutional Review Boards and the Freedom to Take Risks." *New England Journal of Medicine* 307 (18) (28 October 1982): 1156-59.

Rawls, John. "Kantian Constructivism in Moral Theory." *Journal of Philosophy* 77 (September 1980): 515-577.

Rawls, John. "Two Concepts of Rules." Part I, *Philosophical Review* LXIV (1955): 3-13.

Reatig, Natalie. "Can Investigators Appeal Adverse IRB Decisions?" *IRB: A Review of Human Subjects Research* 2 (March 1986): 8-9.

Robertson, John A. "Ethics Committees in Hospitals: Alternative Structures and Responsibilities." *Quality Review Bulletin* 10 (January 1984): 6-10.

Robertson, John A., and Angela R. Holder. "IRB Members and Liability: An Exchange of Views." *IRB: A Review of Human Subjects Research* 2 (2) (January 1980): 10-11.

Roundtree. "The Anguish of Peer Review." *Journal of the Medical Association of Georgia* 67 (April 1978): 287.

Self, Donnie J., and Joy D. Skeel. "Potential Roles of the Medical Ethicist in the Clinical Setting." *Theoretical Medicine* 7 (1) (February 1986): 33-39.

Shapiro, Samuel. "The Decison to Publish Ethical Dilemmas." *Journal of Chronic Diseases* 38 (4) (1985): 365-72.

Shimberg, Benjamin. "The Relationship Among Accreditation, Certification and Licensure." *Federation Bulletin* 71 (4) (April 1984): 99-116.

Siegler, Mark. "Ethics Committees: Decision by Bureaucracy." *Hastings Center Report* 16 (5) (June 1986): 22-24.

Schoeman, Ferdinand D. "On Incapacitating the Dangerous." *Philosophical Quarterly* 16 (1) (1979).

Sugarman, Stephen D. "Doing Away with Tort Law." *California Law Review* 73 (1985): 555-664.

Taylor, Richard. "Causation." *Monist* 47 (1963): 287- 313.

Thompson, Paul B. "Collective Responsibility and Professional Roles." *Journal of Business Ethics* 5 (1986): 151-54.

Toulmin, Stephen. "How Medicine Saved the Life of Ethics." *Perspectives in Biology and Medicine* 25 (4) (Summer 1982): 736-50.

Twiss, Summer R., Jr. "The Problem of Moral Responsibility in Medicine." *Journal of Medicine and Philosophy* 2 (4) (December 1977): 330-75.

Veatch, Robert M. "Liability and the IRB Member: The Ethical Aspects." *IRB: A Review of Human Subjects Research* 1(3) (May 1979): 8-9.

Veatch, Robert M. "Patients' Rights and Physician Accountability: Problems with PSROs." *Bioethics Quarterly* 3 (3/4) (Fall/Winter 1981): 137-55.

Walters, LeRoy, edited by "Bioethics Commissions: International Perspectives." *Journal of Medicine and Philosophy* 14 (4) (August 1989) (Special Issue).

Woodward, William E. "An Investigator/Defendant Corrects the Record." *IRB: A Review of Human Subject Research* 1 (4) (August/September 1979): 10.

Woolf, Patricia K. "Ensuring Integrity in Biomedical Publication." *Journal of the American Medical Association* 258 (23) (18 December 1987).

Newspaper and Newsletter Articles

Cook-Deegan, Robert Mullan. "Abortion Politics Deals Death Blow to Bioethics Body Set Up by Congress." *Kennedy Institute of Ethics Newsletter* IV (3) (3 July 1990): 3, 5, 2.

"Focus on Medical Specialists: Credentialing the Superspecialist." *Staff Privileges Report* III (3) (July 1990): 5-6.

Health Policy Week. 19 (24) (25 June 1990): 1, 3.

Hinz, Christine A. "West Virginia Ruling Shields Some Peer Review Activities: Court Orders Opening of Disciplinary Records." *American Medical Association News*, 16 December 1986.

Hornblower, Margot. "Baby M: Battle of 'Class and Gender.'" *Washington Post.* 17 February 1987, p. A4, col. 1.

Malcolm, Andrew H. "Medical Ethicists Are a New Source of Second Opinion." *New York Times*, 20 July 1986, p. E24.

Otten, Alan L. "Ethics Experts Help More Doctors Handle Hard Moral Decisions." *The Wall Street Journal*, 6 March 1987, p. 1.

Official Documents and Regulations

American Hospital Association. General Council Special Committee on Biomedical Ethics. *Values in Conflict: Resolving Ethical Issues in Hospital Care*. Chicago: American Hospital Association, 1985.

American Hospital Association. *Guidelines: Hospital Committees on Biomedical Ethics*. Chicago: American Hospital Association, 1984.

American Medical Association, Judicial Council. "Guidelines for Ethics Committees in Health Care Institutions." *Journal of the American Medical Association* 253 (18) (10 May 1985): 2698-99.

Breaden, Dale G., and Bryant L. Galusha. "Official 1985 Federation Summary of Reported Disciplinary Actions." *Federation Bulletin*. Federation of State Medical Boards of the United States, Inc. (October 1986): 300-305.

Committee on Evolving Trends in Society Affecting Life, California Medical Association. "Guidelines for Establishing Bioethics Committees." In *Institutional Ethics Committees and Health Care Decision Making,* edited by Ronald E. Cranford and A. Edward Doudera. 405-11. Ann Arbor, Michigan: Health Administration Press, 1984.

Joint Commission on Accreditation of Hospitals. *1988 AMH: Accreditation Manual for Hospitals*. Chicago, Illinois: Joint Commission on Accreditation of Hospitals, 1987.

President's Commission for the Study of Ethical Problems in Medicine and Biomedical and Behavioral Research. *Deciding to Forego Life-Sustaining Treatment: Ethical, Medical and Legal Issues in Treatment Decisions*. Washington, DC: U.S. Government Printing Office, 1983.

President's Commission for the Study of Ethical Problems in Medicine and Biomedical and Behavioral Research. *IRB Guidebook*. Washington, DC: U.S. Government Printing Office, 1983.

U.S. Congress, House. Representative Sander Levin introducing the Patient Self-Determination Act of 1990. *Congressional Record* (3 April 1990): E943-E944.

U.S. Department of Health, Education and Welfare. *Report on Licensure and Related Personnel Credentialing*. Washington, DC: U.S. Government Printing Office, 1971.

U.S. Department of Health and Human Services. "Ethics Advisory Board; Notice of Establishment." *Federal Register* 53 (12 September 1988): 35232-35233.

U.S. Department of Health and Human Services. "Guidelines for Research Involving Recombinant DNA Molecules." *Federal Register* 51 (7 May 1986): 16958-64.

U.S. Department of Health and Human Services. "Guidelines for Research Involving Recombinant DNA Molecules; Notice." *Federal Register* 51 (7 May 1986): 16958-85.

U.S. Department of Health and Human Services. "Medicare and Medicaid Programs; Changes to Peer Review Organizations Regulations, Proposed Rule." *Federal Register* 53 (16 March 1988): 8654-67.

U.S. Department of Health and Human Services. "Medicare and Medicaid Programs; Utilization and Quality Control Peer Review Organization (PRO) Assumption of Medicare Review Functions and Coordination with Medicaid, Final Rule." *Federal Register* 50 (17 April 1985): 15312-74.

U.S. Department of Health and Human Services. "Service and Treatment for Disabled Infants; Model Guidelines for Health Care Providers To Establish Infant Care Review Committees." *Federal Register* 51 (15 April 1985): 14893-900.

U.S. Office of Science and Technology Policy of the Executive Office of the President. "Proposed Model Federal Policy for Protection of Human Subjects; Response to the First Biennial Report of the President's Commission for the Study of Ethical Problems in Medicine and Biomedical and Behavioral Research. *Federal Register* 51 (3 June 1986): 20204-17.

Unpublished Papers

Howe, Edmund G. "When Physicians Impose Values on Patients: An Ethics Consultant's Responsibilities." A paper contributed to a conference co-sponsored by the National Institutes of Health and the University of California at San Francisco, 7-8 October 1985.

McCarthy, Charles R. "Ethics Consultation in the Context of Federal Regulations to Protect Human Subjects of Research." A presentation at a conference cosponsored by the National Institutes of Health and the University of California at San Francisco, 7-8 October 1985.

Moreno, Jonathan D. "Ethics by Committee: The Moral Authority of Consensus." A paper presented at the Kennedy Institute of Ethics, Washington, DC, 11 November 1987.

Rothenberg, Leslie Steven. "Clinical Ethicists and Hospital Ethics Consultants: The Nature and Desirability of Their 'Clinical' Role." A paper contributed to a conference cosponsored by the National Institutes of Health and the University of California at San Francisco, 7-8 October 1985.

Cases
Cruzan v. Director, Missouri Department of Health, US, 110 S. Ct. 2841 (1990).

Francis v. United Jersey Bank, 432 A.2d 814 (NJ 1981).

Graham v. Allis-Chalmers Manufacturing Co., 188 A.2d125 (DE 1963).

In re Quinlan, 355 A.2d 647 (N.J. 1976), *cert. denied*, 429 US 922.

Litwin (Rosemarin) v. Allen, 25 N.Y.S.2d 667 (Sup. Ct. 1940).

United States v. Alvarez, 610 F.2d 1250 (5th Cir. 1980).

Webster v. Reproductive Health Services, US , 109 S. Ct. 3040 (1989).

Statutes
Alabama Code. Sec. 22-2-1 (1984).

Arizona Revised Statutes Annotated. Sec. 36-2404 (1988).

California Civil Code. Sec. 43.7(b) (1982 and 1990 Supplement).

California Evidence Code. Sec. 1157 (1966 and 1990 Supplement).

Federal Food, Drug and Cosmetic Act. 21 USC. secs. 321-392 (1938).

Hawaii Revised Statutes Annotated. Sec. 663-1.7 (1989 Supplement).

Idaho Code. Sec. 54-934 (1988).

Illinois Annotated Statutes. Ch. 110, secs. 8-2101, 8-2103 (Smith-Hurd, 1984 and 1989 Supplement).

Main Revised Statutes Annotated. Tit. 24, sec. 2506 (1988 Supplement).

Maryland Health-General Code Annotated. Secs. 19-306, 19-308, 19-327 (West 1982).

Maryland Health Occupations Code Annotated. Secs. 14-202, 14-601(f) (West 1986).

Massachusetts Annotated Laws. Ch. 111, sec. 203(a)(1988 Supplement).

Minnesota Statute. Sec. 145.63 (West. 1989).

Montana Code annotated. Sec. 37-2-201 (1989).

New Jersey Statutes Annotated. Sec. 2A:84A-22.10 (1990).

New York Education Law. Secs. 6509, 6511 (McKinney, 1985 and 1990 Supplement).

New York Public Health Law. Sec. 30 (McKinney, 1990 Supplement).

Revised Model Business Corporations Act. (1984).

Tennessee Code Annotated. Secs. 63-2, 63-101 to 63-127, 4-507 to 4-527 (1986).

Texas Revised Civil Statutes Annotated. Art. 4447d, sec. 3 (Vernon 1976).

Wisconsin Statutes Annotated. Sec. 15.405(7) (West 1986).